Kate Liber

Herbal Antibiotics and Antivirals

A Complete Guide to Discover the Secrets of Natural Remedies to Prevent and Cure Bacterial and Viral Infections with Medicinal Herbs

Copyright © 2020 publishing.

All rights reserved.

Author: Kate Liberty

No part of this publication may be reproduced, distributed or transmitted in any form or by any means, including photocopying recording or other electronic or mechanical methods or by any information storage and retrieval system without the prior written permission of the publisher, except in the case of brief quotation embodies in critical reviews and certain other non-commercial uses permitted by copyright law.

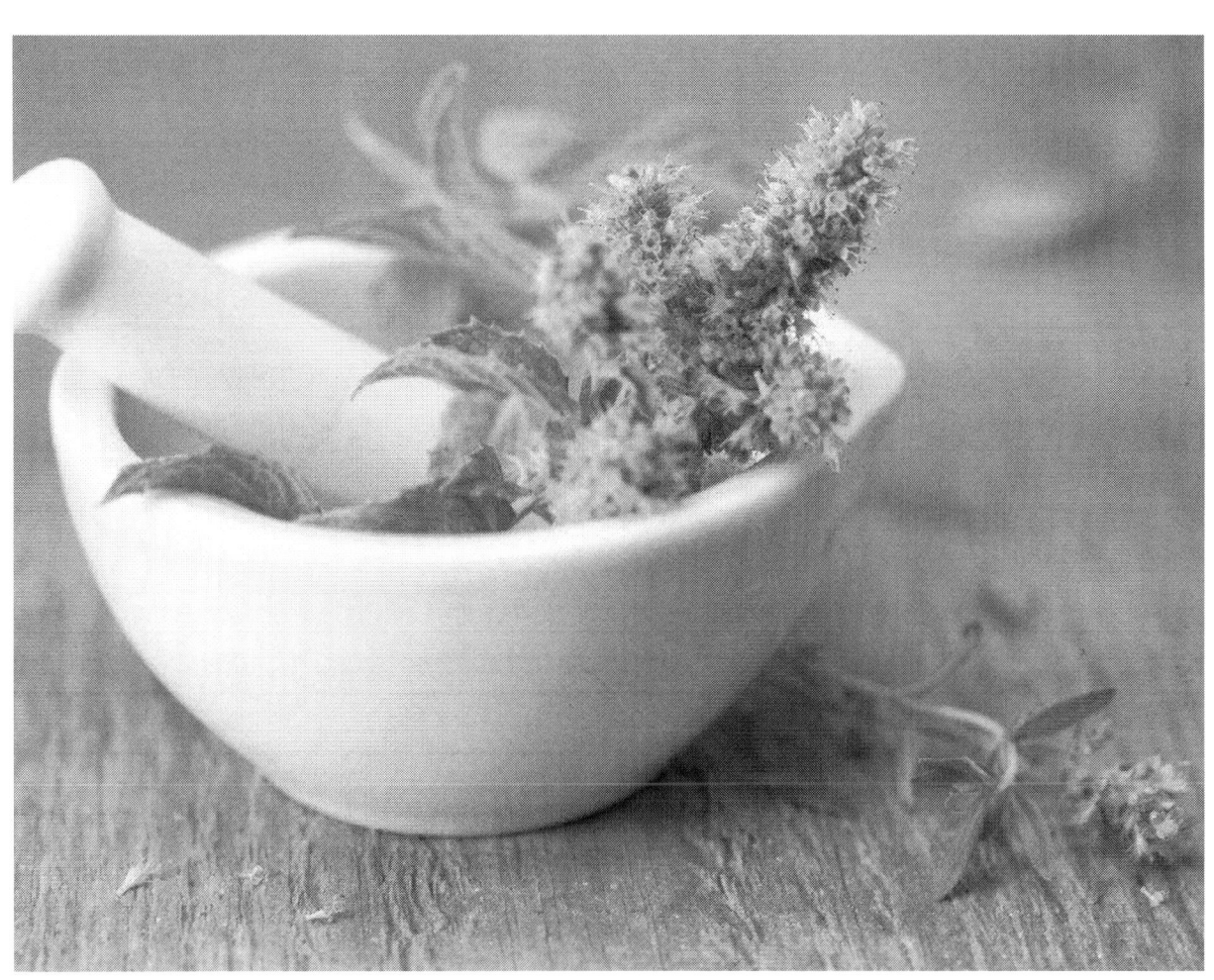

Table of Contents

HERBAL ANTIBIOTICS 6
NATURAL ANTIBIOTICS AND PROBIOTICS 23
HERBAL REMEDIES ARE POWERFUL ANTIBIOTICS 45
ANTIBIOTICS RESISTANCE 48
BREAKING THE ANTIBIOTIC CYCLE 77
HERBAL REMEDIES TO PREVENT ANTIBIOTIC CAUSED SERIOUS ILLNESSES 87
THE IMMUNE SYSTEM 92
NATURAL REMEDIES FOR YEAST INFECTION 107
THE MOST EFFECTIVE HOME REMEDIES FOR URINARY TRACT INFECTION 113
HERBAL ANTIBIOTICS – NATURAL ALTERNATIVES TO SEASONAL SICKNESSES 116
HERBAL ANTIFUNGAL REMEDIES 120
HERBAL HEMORRHOID REMEDIES 124
BV HERBAL REMEDY 126
ANTIVIRAL HERBS 134
THE USE OF ANTIVIRAL DRUGS-ALL YOU NEED TO KNOW 140
HOW HERBAL ANTIVIRAL DRUGS WORK 143
ANTIVIRAL HERBS FOR QUICK AND SAFE RELIEF 147
NATURALLY STRENGTHEN THE IMMUNE SYSTEM WITH ANTIVIRAL HERBS 150
THE BEST SOURCES FOR HERBAL ANTIVIRAL DRUGS 153
COMMON VIRAL INFECTIONS AND THEIR CAUSES 155
COMMON NATURAL ANTIVIRAL HERBS 157

COMMON BACTERIAL INFECTION 163

NATURAL REMEDIES FOR THE TREATMENT OF ALLERGIES 168

TO IMPROVE IMMUNITY, USE PROVEN HERBAL REMEDIES 170

HOW TO USE MEDICINAL HERBS... 172

THE BENEFITS OF GROWING MEDICINAL HERBS...................................... 179

VIRAL INFECTIONS, THE IMMUNE SYSTEM AND ANTIVIRAL SUPPLEMENTS 182

SINUSITIS HERBS 187

EVERYTHING YOU NEED TO KNOW ABOUT HERBS DETOXIFICATION 193

HERBAL ANTIBIOTICS 199

THE PRODUCTION OF MEDICINES 218

HERBAL ANTIBIOTICS

Herbal antibiotics will help build immune reserves and immunodeficiency that optimizes health and quality of life. Herbal mixtures can be effective against drug-resistant bacteria. It has very strong immune activation capabilities as it activates white blood cells to fight bacterial and viral infections. It also activates the production of interferon, a specific protein that protects cells from viral invasion.

The immune system protects against bacteria, viruses, toxins, parasites, and microbes. It is extremely important to maintain a healthy immune system. A poor immune system is more susceptible to infections, colds and flu, cancer, and heart disease. Bacteria live in everything, and hundreds of beneficial bacteria live in the human body, helping to protect against harmful bacteria. Prescription antibiotics are effective in killing bad bacteria, but they also kill good bacteria. Good bacteria are an important part of the immune system, lining the digestive, respiratory, and urinary tract. The use of prescription antibiotics often causes excessive yeast growth, which further weakens the immune system.

Herbs can support good blood chemistry and help purify and detoxify. By nourishing and balancing the system, the body receives what it needs to withstand, repair, and overcome diseases and achieve Optimal Health. Antibiotic herbs are effective for bacterial, viral, and fungal treatment. Treatment may not be faster than medications. Although antibiotic herbs are milder than pharmaceuticals, they should be taken only if necessary. Prescription antibiotic drugs will always be there when we really need them.

Some Basic Knowledge About Natural Antibiotics

We argue that everyone should have basic knowledge of natural antibiotics. This would include knowledge of natural substances with antibiotic properties and how to use them to achieve this antibiotic effect.

Before delving into our arguments on why we presented that everyone should have basic knowledge about natural antibiotics, it will be essential for us to give a brief introduction to the concept of antibiotics in general and, in particular, to the natural antibiotics.

Now, antibiotics are substances used in the fight against bacteria. Bacteria, as we all know, are among the microbes (therefore mainly fungi and viruses) that cause us diseases. Probably, there are more diseases attributable to bacteria than to any other type of microbes. Not all bacteria cause disease, of course. There are bacteria that are of great help to us, bacteria whose number we try to increase in our body, rather than decimate. But the harmful variety of bacteria must be fought, and the main weapons in this fight are antibiotics.

When antibiotics are synthetically manufactured/formulated in pharmaceutical laboratories, they are called synthetic antibiotics. These synthetic antibiotics are the only types of antibiotics that many of us know about. But the knowledge of natural antibiotics slowly pierces the masses. These natural antibiotics are distinguished from other types of antibiotics by the fact that they are "directly exploited by nature."They are not synthesized in the laboratory. They tend to be just as effective (if to some extent slower to act) as antibiotics that are synthesized in pharmaceutical laboratories. They are considered by many people safer than antibiotics synthesized in laboratories.

Now, there is one of the main reasons why everyone should have a basic knowledge of natural antibiotics: to ensure that in case you have to deal with a bacterial infection in a situation where you don't have access to antibiotics, synthetically produced, they still have a way to cope with the infection. This is important because we know that about some deadly bacterial infections. And while some tasks on their initiative (such as the body's natural immune system eventually overcomes them), most will not be in remission on their own. In fact, when a bacterial disease manifests itself, the presumption is that the body's natural immunity has already been overwhelmed by bacteria. In this case, unless something very drastic happens, it is very unlikely that the body will regain the upper hand over bacteria. Without some kind of mitigation measures (in the form of an antibiotic), the condition in question tends to worsen.

Therefore, within the framework of "survivability" it would be good for everyone to understand natural antibiotics, so that they can distribute them, in the event of a bacterial disease that falls into a situation where they can not access pharmaceutical antibiotics. And since most of the natural antibiotics we are talking about are parts of harmless plants, which strengthen the body's immunity rather than directly kill bacteria, their knowledge (and subsequent regular use), would also be a prudent preventive measure.

Natural Antibiotics Versus Synthetic Antibiotics

We can start with descriptions, in which both reveal substances that are known to help us fight bacteria that can try to harm us. The difference between natural and synthetic antibiotics, however, is that the former are products of nature (directly exploited by the fields, usual parts of plants), while the latter are products of chemical synthesis in the laboratory. To get a synthetic antibiotic, you need to know what chemical combinations have an antibiotic effect (that is, a bactericidal effect), get the chemicals from the ingredients, and mix them in the right proportions to finish with the antibiotic. To obtain a natural antibiotic, on the other hand, you need to know which plants (and which specific parts of them) have an antibiotic effect, and then go out into the fields to get these parts of the plant, using it in the right way and benefit from the said antibiotic effect.

The difference between natural antibiotics and synthetic supplements is not only in terms of definitions, of course.

Natural antibiotics differ from synthetic supplements in terms of speed of work (typical). We tend to see synthetic antibiotics that work faster than natural supplements. But it is necessary to take note of the fact that we are talking about typical cases here: because there are natural antibiotics that are known to work faster than some synthetic supplements. However, the generally faster working speed associated with synthetic antibiotics is the main reason why synthetic supplements are commonly used in medical emergencies; when a person already suffers from a disease emanating from a bacterial infection and where rapid decimation of bacteria is essential. What is remarkable here is that the effectiveness of synthetic antibiotics tends to be their ruin, too, as most of them end up inadvertently killing useful symbiotic bacteria as well.

Natural supplements also differ from synthetic antibiotics in terms of safety profiles. Natural supplements are considered, in general, and in many ways, safer than synthetic antibiotics. It should be noted here, the fact that the use of supplements is not always transient (although it is ideal as it should be). On the contrary, there are people who end up with conditions that require them to use them long-term or very frequently. These people, if they were to use synthetic antibiotics, would almost certainly end up with very unpleasant side effects from this long-term use of antibiotics. But where milder natural supplements are used, the long-term prospects can be much better.

Natural antibiotics differ from synthetic supplements in terms of working mechanisms (typical). We observe a situation where the typical synthetic antibiotic works by directly killing (killing) harmful bacteria and, inevitably, some useful bacteria. This is against a situation where the typical natural antibiotic works not only by killing bacteria but also by improving the body's natural ability to fight such bacterial infections in the future.

Why More and More People Are Resorting To Natural Antibiotics

In recent years, we have seen an ever-increasing number of people opting for the use of natural antibiotics rather than synthetic antibiotics that we trusted so much. It's not that old (that is, natural) antibiotics are a very new invention. These are substances that we have always had from time immemorial. These are practically the substances that our ancestors used to treat and prevent bacterial infections before the pharmaceutical industry approached and offered us the most conveniently available synthetic antibiotics. So, they are not new substances or new discoveries. But their widespread use in recent days is a relatively new phenomenon.

To have a context in which we can understand, we must realize that the human race as we know it today has existed for millions of years (according to the scientific view), or at least thousands of years (according to most religious traditions). In both cases, it is not disputed that the human race has existed for much longer than the pharmaceutical industry. It is also very little disputed that most of the bacteria that are harmful to us today were still harmful to our ancestors. And it is in light of these facts that we have just appreciated the other fact of the effect that antibiotics are not a recent invention. They were always there; these are the substances that our ancestors, until the relatively recent development of the pharmaceutical industry, used to cope with the above-mentioned antibacterial infections.

With the advent of the pharmaceutical industry, natural antibiotics were almost forgotten. The pharmaceutical industry, after all, presented us with antibiotics that were mercilessly effective and that was conveniently available (like pills that you could just pop and get almost instant relief).

This has been the status quo for many years to the extent that, as mentioned above, people have virtually forgotten the natural antibiotics they had used before the arrival of those with synthetic formulations.

Then something happened only a few years ago, people began to think again about natural antibiotics, and many began to use them rather than synthetic antibiotics. What interests us in research are the reasons for this change.

Apparently, the greatest attraction for natural antibiotics is their safety. For many years, fears about the safety of synthetic antibiotics have been expressed. Of course, they have always been mercilessly effective. But it was also pointed out that their ruthless effectiveness had a great cost to those who used it. Antibiotics would leave many long-term side effects. And in an attempt to help us decimate harmful bacteria, most of them tended to destroy useful bacteria in our body, leaving us with a new set of health problems. In addition, our bodies tended to develop resistance to them (after recognizing them for the "unnatural" foreign entities they were). This is largely what brought people back to natural antibiotics, which are much safer (most of them are food substances and herbs that we otherwise use day after day, if only for different reasons). Our bodies seem to cope better with them. And natural antibiotics are also much cheaper than synthetic antibiotics.

The Two Main Working Mechanism for Natural Antibiotics

There are two main mechanisms by which natural antibiotics work. Before venturing out to explore the exact nature of these two mechanisms, it will be good to indicate to us briefly the concept of antibiotics in general and natural antibiotics. That would serve several purposes. It would be useful for the uninitiated (those of us who encounter these problems for the first time). And this would lay a conceptual basis for understanding the recently explored working mechanisms.

An antibiotic is almost everything that kills bacteria. This is one of the reasons why a person would like to kill bacteria: when these bacteria turn out to be harmful to their interests. In most cases, we examine the bacteria that cause our diseases. The range of diseases caused by bacteria is wide, some are minor diseases, with which most of us live, and others are really a serious illness (such as tuberculosis), which are fatal in nature. By extension, the term antibiotic may also refer to a substance that weakens the effects of harmful bacteria in the body, and a substance that boosts the body's natural ability to fight bacteria. Because it turned out that our body is constantly in contact with harmful bacteria, with which we fight antibiotics. However, until it is our immunity as strong as should be, are these bacteria easily repelled by our body naturally, without any help. Sometimes, however, the natural immunity of our body is impaired, or presented to a bacterial infection, which simply cannot avoid, and this leads to disease, which can usually be overcome with the use of antibiotics.

The antibiotic can be natural or synthetic. The first is an antibiotic obtained "naturally," unlike the second, which is synthesized in the lab by mixing different strengths of chemicals. A typical natural antibiotic will be a substance obtained from a part of the plant.

As mentioned above, there are two main mechanisms by which these natural antibiotics work.

The first mechanism by which the natural antibiotics act is to decimate (directly) offending bacteria. In this case, the antibiotic in question will simply be a deadly substance for bacteria. When you take a natural antibiotic, it eventually finds its way into the bloodstream, where the offending bacteria is likely to have a day in the field."The bacteria eventually come into contact with it and die. Then a person is cured of the disease it caused.

The second mechanism by which natural antibiotics improve the body's ability to repel bacteria. As mentioned above, when the bacterial population will start to grow to a level where they can cause disease, it tends to be the result of the failure of the natural immunity of our body. In such cases, there would be a chance to achieve better (and more sustainable) results by strengthening the body's natural ability to fight with bacteria and other microbes that may try to harm you.

Tips for Treating Bacterial Infections:

General recommendations for infection: eliminate caffeine, alcohol, sugar, refined foods, meat, and dairy products while you have an acute infection. Eat lightly. Drink a lot of warm and Atmospheric drinks like herbal tea. Juice fasting or even water for a few days can be very useful during infection. Enemas can help rinse the system. It is recommended that vitamin C, beta-carotene, and zinc strengthen the immune system. Herbs like Echinacea and Hydrastis (hydrast of Canada) can help support the immune system, but more specific, herbs are often more useful. Saunas and steam baths can also be useful for detoxifying the system during infections. Massage can accelerate the removal of toxins, in particular, foot massage with garlic oil. Listen to what your body is trying to tell you and ask what it needs. Stay! When you are sick, do not go beyond your limits. Recovery can take twice as long.

Throat Infection: even if you suffer from streptococcal angina (diagnosed by throat culture), natural therapies can be very useful, but it is important to check a blood test, that no streptococci persist, because, on occasion, an unobserved streptococcal infection can lead to kidney, joint or heart problems. Throat infections often respond well to garglings, such as saltwater, Calendula, Canadian Hydra, myrrh, or bitter orange oil. There are many excellent herbal remedies available for the throat. Homeopathy works very well for throat infection. We often use Belladonna, Lachesis, Lycopodium, Phytolacca, and Mercurius for sore throat. Streptococcal angina can also be treated with a very unusual drug, spigelia, with complete pain relief within two days.

Skin Infections: a mixture of tincture and St. John's wort is what we use for bacterial skin infections. Other commonly used herbs are Canadian Hydra, comfrey, and plantain. Bubbles and cysts can be successfully treated with hot compresses, Ginger compresses, and Epsom salt dips, and homeopathic remedies such as silica and Heparsulphuris. Fungal infections often respond well, even to homeopathy or the application of diluted vinegar. Turmeric powder and tea oil are also effective.

Bladder Infection: a word of caution with bladder infection, treat them immediately. The longer you wait, the more pain and a greater risk of kidney infection and end up with antibiotics. We recommend plenty of water, cranberry juice or capsules, herbs (usually Hydrastis, bearberry, Bucchu, Chimaphilia, Berberis, and others) and homeopathy (such remedies as Staphysagria, Cantharis, Apis and Sarsaparilla, to name a few).

Breast Infection: remember, no dairy products! Drink plenty of hot ginger tea. To break the mucus, we use an excellent Ayurvedic combination called Sitopalades. Homeopathic remedies such as Kali bichromicum, Pulsatilla, Mercurius, Natrum muriaticum, and Allium cepa work well.

NATURAL ANTIBIOTICS AND PROBIOTICS

If you have ever been bitten by a wild animal, have a bad cut, or maybe it was the unfortunate recipient of sexually transmitted diseases, most likely, your friendly doctor will prescribed antibiotics. Antibiotics are drugs that kill or slow down the growth of bacteria. Penicillin and amoxicillin are two commonly prescribed antibiotics.

The problem with synthetic antibiotics is the ability of the human body to become resistant to these drugs. Every time you take antibiotics, your body will create more tolerance. Therefore, taking antibiotics for any disease related to the bacteria it catches, weakens the body's ability to fight infections. The good news is that there are ways to prevent infection and boost your immune system without these drugs!

Long before Alexander Fleming, Nobel laureate, bacteriologist, discovered these antibacterial drugs that naturally existed in a variety of foods and herbs. Natural antibiotics and antimicrobial substances are found mainly in onion and garlic, herbs, honey, sauerkraut, and fermented foods such as unpasteurized raw sauerkraut, raw pickles, and probiotic yogurt. All these dishes increase the immune system and have antibiotic properties. These foods promote healthy digestion and help your body defend against infectious diseases.

Foods with a high content of vitamin C, such as cabbage, oranges and citrus fruits, tomatoes, papaya, sweet pepper, and kiwi, have great natural antibiotic immunostimulant properties. These fruits and vegetables are rich in antioxidants, which help protect cells from free radicals (unstable molecules) that can cause cancer.

Raw cabbage, raw cucumbers, and probiotic yogurt contain good microorganisms that help digest. This good bacterium replaces bad bacteria in the intestine, provides additional defense against infection. A diet rich in these types of foods will help you fight bad bacteria and improve your health and well-being in general.

What about the onions and garlic you're asking for? Onions and garlic contain natural antibacterial properties in the form of sulfur compounds. These compounds are used as an anti-inflammatory and protect the body from colds and flu.

Honey natural antibiotic properties were discovered long before doctors created prescribed medications. Honey has a natural enzyme that releases hydrogen peroxide into the body. Hydrogen peroxide has the ability to stop the growth of various types of bacteria that could otherwise spread and cause disease.

Herbs such as aloe, licorice, and almost all other herbs, you can think that they have good antibacterial properties that will help in the fight against infections. Aloe is commonly applied to cuts, falls, and burns to ensure faster healing and prevent bacterial infections. It is also active against herpes simplex type 1 and type 2. Licorice acts against streptococci, E-coli, staphylococcal infection, and even tuberculosis.

All these natural antibiotics, if they are incorporated into your daily diet, will support a strong immune system. When your body needs a little backup to fight an army of bacteria, consuming these foods will help defend your body. So, the next time you feel cold, scratch your knee or engrave your hand on it, such as a dinner pot, to get a natural antibiotic to help a speedy recovery!

The Natural Antibiotic and Antimicrobial Wonder

We live in a time when pathogens are becoming increasingly resistant to antibiotic therapy. Many of these diseases become serious killers, such as MRSA or methicillin-resistant Staphylococcus aureus, vancomycin-resistant worm, or Enterococcus, and mycobacteria or tuberculosis. Resistance is the ability of a microorganism to resist the effects of antibiotics. This resistance occurs in nature through the process of natural selection, but it can also occur when "evolutionary" stress is applied to a certain population of microorganisms as with overuse or misuse of antibiotic therapy.

The result is an increase in the number of organisms that have become resistant, some of them to more than one antibiotic. These are the so-called "super bacteria." Inaddition, the strongest antibiotics used to kill these "super bacteria" can have undesirable side effects on the human population. In some cases, these side effects can be harmful, such as the disease being treated. There is a solution to the problem that is almost ignored by modern medicine, especially in the United States. However, this solution is beginning to gain popularity around the world, especially in the holistic communities of Health and alternative medicine and in countries with less bureaucracy to stop the progress of natural and non-pharmacological therapies. This solution is the use of a colloidal silver solution, a real natural antibiotic.

The colloidal silver solution is a liquid suspension of microscopic silver particles, particles of colloidal importance that remain in suspension without forming a dissolved or ionic solution. Colloidal silver is a known, powerful antimicrobial agent. Concentrations of five parts per million have been found to kill many infectious bacteria. Its mechanism of action appears to be through the oligodynamic effect by inhibiting the expression of enzymes and other proteins essential to produce ATP or adenosine-5'-triphosphate. It is toxic to several resistant organisms such as MRSA and tuberculosis, and some recent studies have also shown an effect against viruses such as influenza A, the virus that causes influenza in humans.

In the United States, companies that produce or sell a colloidal silver solution are prohibited by the FDA from claiming any therapeutic value of the product. It cannot be labeled as a natural antibiotic, even if that is really what it is. The agency allows you to label and sell as a food supplement until drug applications are submitted. Ongoing scientific studies have been conducted by many independent laboratories to validate the effectiveness of this potential antimicrobial Marvel, and colloidal silver has been tested against several resistant and non-resistant pathogens with good results. It has been approved by the EPA for use as a disinfectant in hospitals and medical clinics in the United States. Silver is also used in the treatment of burns and bedsores.

Internationally, however, the story is very different. Many countries have recognized and used this powerful agent, this natural antibiotic, to treat several pathogenic pathogens. Colloidal silver solution is widely used successfully in African hospitals to treat malaria, cholera, AIDS, influenza, hepatitis, respiratory infections such as pneumonia and bronchitis, tuberculosis, gonorrhea, sinus infections, food poisoning, vaginitis, staphylococcal infections and streptococci, Thrush, burns, wounds and skin infections. This author used it effectively against breast infections, peritoneal infections, dental infections, cuts, and wounds.

It seems that there is no end to the beneficial effects of this extraordinary metal. I think of the great sculptor

George Washington and his research on peanuts. Colloidal silver solution could be the antimicrobial wonder the world desperately needs, as more and more of these antibiotic-resistant super insects are popping up every day. We can only hope that American medicine will reach the rest of the world and start using colloidal money against these enemies of our health. If you want to know more about this amazing miracle "metal" this powerful natural antibiotic, or if you want to share with me your thoughts, pro or with, do not hesitate to contact me. I'd like to discuss this with you in person.

Side Effects of Synthetic Antibiotics

Synthetic antibiotics are increasingly ineffective against bacteria. However, antibiotics still develop some unfortunate side effects, which can be avoided with the use of antibiotic herbs.

1. Vaginal Yeast Infection

As already mentioned in the previous section, the use of synthetic antibiotics effectively removes all "good" bacteria from the digestive tract. As good bacteria move from the gastrointestinal tract, yeast can begin to develop by crawling into the vaginal and digestive Arena. This imbalance between bacteria and yeast leads to yeast infection. Yeast infection includes such embarrassing and unpleasant elements as redness, swelling, itching, and burning in the vaginal area. 2013 antibiotic study showed that twenty-five percent of all women who took synthetic antibiotics, in fact, developed a yeast infection.

2. Nausea, vomiting, and diarrhea

Each digestive tract must maintain a good dose of good and bad bacteria to form good digestion. Synthetic antibiotics disrupt this balance and cause diarrhea. According to a recent study, about fifteen percent of all antibiotic users have antibiotic-related diarrhea.

3. Drug Interaction

The company's constant demand for more and more drugs can lead to interactions between different drugs. Side effects that result from these interactions include headache, stomach pain, and other serious health problems. In addition, other synthetic antibiotics can effectively reduce the body's ability to function properly. An example is the use of some oral contraceptives. Other synthetic antibiotics can prevent contraception and lead to an unplanned pregnancy. It is important that people keep a constant dialogue with doctors about the drugs they use to ensure proper functioning.

4. Hypersensitivity or induced allergens

Several patients report allergic reactions to synthetic drugs they take. According to a 2011 study, about 32% of cases of drug allergy were caused by antibiotics. These allergens are physically observed on the skin, with the appearance of rashes or urticaria.

Other rare side effects include kidney stones, sensitivity to the sun, a sense of hearing loss, and occasional changes in blood clotting.

The current crisis of synthetic antibiotics

The media accused him of all the speakers. The world is in the midst of an antibiotic crisis. Bacteria are increasingly resistant to synthetic antibiotics that doctors throw at them, leading to the latest new outbreak of bacteria. As each new bacterium evolves, new synthetic drugs must be developed to compete with them. How, exactly, is it possible so quickly? Essentially, bacteria are among the most adaptable organisms on the planet. Their reproduction rate is only twenty minutes - whereas humans usually wait twenty years before reproducing. In addition, each reproduction leads to a new evolution. These new strains of bacteria can also teach other strains of bacteria how to build against other strains. And how long can it last? The medical world understands that the days of synthetic antibiotics are coming to an end. People need to start preparing for this sudden future.

One of the reasons for this antibiotic crisis appeared because doctors abused and over-diagnosed seemingly "miraculous" antibiotics for several years. Penicillin, the miraculous antibiotic that erased countless diseases in the middle of the 20th century, provides an excellent example of this over diagnosis. It was discovered in 1942; however, less than half a century later, forty million pounds of penicillin was used in the United States each year. Today, more than sixty million pounds of penicillin are used every year, eventually becoming useless in the next century due to its excessive use. Bacteria, as mentioned above, can be formulated against this onslaught of antibiotics. Soon, this excessive use of penicillin will certainly lead to a tragedy because bacteria act against the drug.

In addition, research shows that synthetic antibiotics enter and leave the body generally unchanged. This means that they work through the digestive system and in the world's largest "water" without altering it. After the water is cleaned by groundwater processes, the water still maintains low levels of this antibiotic "rejection."Therefore, even if people drink ordinary water, they still build a small resistance toothier antibiotics. Ultimately, these antibiotics will not work effectively on these people because the bacteria in their body already understand how to work against it.

Of course, curbing the use of synthetic antibiotics in today's culture proves difficult with the mentality of society. People want to eliminate their diseases immediately, and who can blame them? No one wants to feel terrible. No one wants to lose their lives because of the disease. Synthetic antibiotics are invaluable because they act quickly. They are powerful in all life-threatening disease situations. However, society must limit their use of these synthetic antibiotics and reserve these antibiotics for life-threatening scenarios. It is necessary to limit the antibiotics of the recent attack on the environment, thanks to the water supply. In addition, these antibiotics should be eliminated in their use to strengthen the strength and health of farm animals. Synthetic antibiotics have a purpose and were created for a reason. However, these reasons have been stretched to cover almost the whole world, making them almost useless in the years to come.

In addition, with each dose of synthetic antibiotics, the immune system of people immediately begins to break. The immune system is an amazing mechanism that initially allows a person to slowly refute the attacks of bacteria. However, synthetic antibiotics actually penetrate the body and kill both good and bad bacteria. They kill, for example, the undeniably important flora of the digestive tract. This removal of the flora can lead to yeast infections and unpleasant sensations in the stomach. Remember that the body needs continuous defense against constant attacks, and the elimination of these good bacteria first creates a tasteless environment in which you can immediately become sicker.

Synthetic antibiotics require a specific "course" for people to follow. When, for example, a person starts an antibiotic but does not complete the established course, the person leaves live heavy bacteria in his system. This remaining bacteria actually works to regenerate to the "next generation" of surviving bacteria, thus having the ability to be resistant to the very antibiotics that could have killed them.

The antibiotic crisis creates a vicious circle of stronger drugs, stronger bacteria, and weaker immune systems. People need to start turning to the ultimate rewards of using herbal antibiotics in order to escape the cycle and feed towards better overall health.

Common Natural Antiviral Herbs

There are hundreds of herbs that are known to show a significant amount of antiviral activity when used. They can be easily accessible in your garden or the local market, while others can be very difficult to find. It is advisable to consult an expert on herbal products, to get the right dosage and conditions of use. For example, some herbs should not be taken during pregnancy. Also, realize that most of the indicated herbs are used to treat more than one viral infection. Some are also strong enough to kill all other harmful pathogens. It is also possible to find an infection that has more than one natural remedy.

Olive leaf can be used in tea with mint or as a capsule. Most often, it is used in the treatment of influenza, colds, and herpes.

Balm on Lemon Leaves is another herb rich in antiviral properties. It is used in the treatment of gastric diseases and skin infections when applied locally. For oral administration, it is possible to make an infusion (add warm water). It is believed that it is not suitable for use during pregnancy.

Adding ginger to tea and meals not only makes it tastier, but it is also known to prevent and reduce the time it takes for the disappearance of colds. It also relieves pain in the neck and chest. When mixed with honey, it is a strong herb in the treatment of influenza and the reduction of sore throat. It can also be crushed or cut into small pieces and added to hot water.

Chlorella is a small unicellular green alga, which is not only an impressive source of nutrition but also known to improve the immune system. A strong immune system helps fight viruses, thereby preventing infection or preventing the spread of infection.

Chamomiles are used to make herbal infusions for medical purposes. This daisy-like plant is used to treat gastrointestinal disorders and relieve inflammation and ulcers. Preference is given to the removal of crushed juice, which is added to hot water.

Cayenne pepper is undoubtedly one of the most powerful herbs in the world. It has many medicinal properties; it is the treatment and relief of colds, sore throats, stomach pain, and prevent the emergence of other pathogens, such as fungi. It is added to food as a spice.

Cranberry is not only used for its culinary activities; it is, in fact, a strong medicinal plant. It is used to treat disorders that occur in the gastrointestinal tract and circulatory complications. Fruit juice is drunk in a full or half-full cup. It's sweet, so you do not need to add sweetener, as in the case of other herbs.

The weed, commonly known as black-bunched Acea, is used to treat kidney infections and sore throats. The grass is squeezed and drunk for a few days to see its effects. However, the herb has serious side effects, such as dizziness, headache, cramps, nausea, vomiting, sweating, and low blood pressure.

Chili has been used in traditional medicine for centuries, especially in Asian countries like India. It is used to treat herpes and other respiratory infections. It is used in food or applied locally by adding water or milk and is one of the most commonly used spices in the world.

Garlic is an indisputable traditional medicine. It is used as a remedy for various diseases, including warts, influenza, and colds. There are other natural ways to treat genital warts, for example, take oat baths or put slices of onions on warts. However, the onion is not scientifically proven enough. I advise you to consult a doctor because these drugs treat only warts, not HPV, which caused warts. They say that chewing raw garlic helps patients with high blood pressure. Most people use garlic as a dish, although it leaves a smell that does not disappear easily.

Astragalus Root is used as a preventive measure against influenza. It works best by increasing the body's immune system, which allows the body to fight viruses. It is recommended to use it in advance flu season, not when you already have it. Use it in herbal tea or cooked in food.

Cat bile, taken in capsule form or in tea, is a strong antiviral, antibacterial and antifungal plant. It is also a powerful stimulant of the immune system.

We cannot talk about herbs without mentioning aloe vera. It is a plant that heals almost everything. It is from the same family as the agave. It is very bitter and may require an additional sweetener; preference is given to honey. It can be administered orally or locally and is considered very effective.

The roots, leaves, seeds, and berries of the elderberry tree are used to treat colds and flu. Due to the high level of cyanide present in the plant, it is necessary to boil completely before using it as a medicine.

Oregano oil is used as a medicine and flavor in food. It is a powerful antiviral, as it accelerates the healing process and prevents irritation of the skin when applied locally.

Licorice root is used as tea and drunk alone or can be mixed with other herbal teas in the treatment of stomach ulcers. It is both antibacterial and antiviral.

Most of the bacteria present in the human body are not harmful; on the contrary, they are very beneficial. It is estimated that only 1% of bacteria in our bodies are harmful. The rest is useful for facilitating digestion and other important functions of the body. Some bacteria are also known to prevent cancer risks and help in the respiratory and urinary tract.

Unlike viruses, bacteria are living microorganisms that can live and reproduce by itself, without attaching himself to a living cell. They are also larger than viruses.

Common Bacterial Infections

It is widely known that not all bacteria are harmless and beneficial; some are very harmful and can have a significant impact on human health. Some of these infections include tuberculosis, which affects millions of people, especially in sub-Saharan Africa. It is very contagious and scattered in the air. It affects the respiratory system, including the lungs, and could kill if not detected and treated in time.

Among other common bacterial infections include typhoid, tetanus, syphilis, pneumonia, Hansen's disease, cavities, gingivitis, epiglottitis, Tonsillitis, Legionnaires disease, whooping cough, anthrax, and meningitis.

There are bacteria transmitted through unprotected sexual intercourse. These include syphilis, chlamydia, and gonorrhea. These infections are treatable. Timely detection and treatment are recommended to prevent other complications, such as pelvic inflammatory disease.

Prostatitis is a bacterial infection that affects the prostate in men. In women, some bacteria can cause urinary tract infections.

Home natural antibiotics

Antibiotics can also be called antibacterial drugs. Pharmaceutical antibiotics come from certain types of fungi. They are used to treat and treat bacterial infections. People who abuse antibiotics are known to develop resistance; this means that medicines, when taken, can't work.

Most of the pharmaceutical antibiotics prescribed by doctors may show signs of side effects such as nausea, dizziness, and vomiting, while some cause allergic reactions such as skin rash or itching; some may also kill the good bacteria that help with some of the functions in the body. We can't rule out side effects when using natural substances; if, however, any and most of them are manageable, there are fewer side effects.

There are millions of people who are allergic to certain herbs; some people are allergic to nuts, others to honey, and others can be allergic to berries. One of the advantages of using natural remedies is that it is common to find more than one natural treatment for an infection. In this case, you can choose one; you are not allergic. Let's look at some common natural antibiotics and infections that heal.

Garlic and onions have been used for their antibacterial and antiviral abilities since time immemorial. They suspect that they help reduce inflammation and reduce the risk of hypertension and stroke.

It has been proven that any food rich in vitamin C, contains antibacterial and antiviral properties. They stimulate the body's immunity, which allows the body to defend itself and accelerate healing. The main sources of vitamin C are fruits such as strawberries, lemons and limes, pineapple, melons and oranges, and most of the vegetables, such as broccoli, tomatoes, spinach, cabbage, and cabbage. Kiwi is not only rich in vitamin C, but it should also contain all other essential nutrients. It is the best fruit for all nutrients, and also one of the most expensive fruits.

Eucalyptus produces a powerful antiseptic that kills most pathogens, including bacteria. It is added to tea and gives a wonderful taste.

Some bacteria are transmitted through the food we eat. The use of horseradish in the food you eat. Bacteria are killed even before they enter the body. It is used as a vegetable.

Coconut oil contains an important substance known as lauric acid. Its main function is to dissolve pathogens. Oil can be used in the preparation of dishes, or oil can be consumed alone.

Scientists have suggested using fermented foods such as fermented vegetables to help give the body the right bacteria. These foods are known as probiotics and are recommended for use with antibiotics.

It is known that the root of Marshmallow has analgesic properties. It is also effective for killing bacteria in the urinary tract. It is best to take it orally in the form of infusion (with warm water). Another plant that can be used to treat urinary tract infections is Yarrow. It is also used as tea. It is not recommended to use it during pregnancy, as it can cause uterine contractions.

Turmeric is a very strong medicinal plant, which is usually ground to form a yellow/orange powder. It is used to treat various infections, including bacterial, fungal, and viral infections.

HERBAL REMEDIES ARE POWERFUL ANTIBIOTICS

If you are seriously ill, do you take this medicine? Do you want to take herbal remedies? Or will you choose prescription drugs?

Before you decide which of the two options is best for you, I advise you to continue reading.

If we compare the effectiveness of herbal remedies and prescription drugs, we wonder which one is the most powerful. Some people have doubts about herbal remedies because they consider plants less effective than medicines. Herbalists responded that herbs are gifts of nature to mankind. God created nature so that herbal remedies came from God. So who do you think is more powerful? Is it God or man?

Antibiotics have been hailed as man's "greatest breakthrough" in the field of medicine. The purpose of antibiotics to kill bacteria or germs that may be the cause of our diseases. But what most of the human population is not aware of are the dangerous side effects of antibiotics.

Yes, antibiotics can kill bad bacteria and good bacteria. They kill toxic germs in our bloodstream. The sad news is that even healthy bacteria, white flakes, end. After seven days of taking antibiotics, there are still inside us, bad bacteria that can multiply in large numbers and soon become toxic germs and could hurt us a lot. We become depressed, tired, and prone to various respiratory diseases.

Recent studies show that prescription drugs have more horrible side effects than herbal remedies.

According to the research, Paxil should not be given to patients who have suicidal tendencies, as this can only worsen the patient's condition. Viagra is also on the list of drugs with harmful side effects. The causes of blindness.

It may be good advice to take acidophilus after undergoing treatment with antibiotics prescribed by your doctor. They say acidophilus capsules contain billions of healthy bacteria. Also, a good source of acidophilus is yogurt and grapefruit seed extract pills.

But most importantly, take oregano.

Herbalists argue that oregano is the most powerful antibiotic in nature. As an effective herbal remedy, oregano has been clinically proven to kill bad bacteria that the strongest prescribed antibiotic cannot eliminate.

Oregano comes in the form of oil or capsules. This can be taken orally or mixed with grapefruit juice.

Another important aspect of oregano is that it does not kill white flakes, but rather promotes their growth and kills Black weeds.

If taken regularly, oregano treats sinusitis, asthma, bronchitis, emphysema, and other respiratory diseases or allergies.

So,it's up to you. Depending on the chosen drug, always keep in mind that your actions and the consequences of these actions are your responsibility. Make sure these do not endanger other humans and yourself—better prevention than cure.

ANTIBIOTICS RESISTANCE

Antibiotic resistance is a form of drug resistance, in which bacteria can survive after exposure to one or more antibiotics. These become known as "multi drug Resistant"(MDR) or, more commonly" Superbugs." The most famous of these superbugs is MRSA (methicillin-resistant Staphylococcus aureus).

Drug resistance of superbugs can be caused by mutation or acquisition of resistant genes from other bacteria. However, it can also be laid on the wide use of antibiotics. Our bodies are so accustomed to them that they no longer have the desired effect on our immune system.

AMR = antimicrobial resistance

30. April 2018, the World Health Organization report issued the following recommendations on how to combat antibiotic resistance:

Taking antibiotics only if prescribed by a doctor.

Complete the entire cycle of antibiotics, even if you feel better.

Never share antibiotics with other people or use the remaining recipes.

While the abuse of antibiotics is an important factor of bacteria resistant to medication, there are other things that you can do every day to prevent this.

Before and after handling food, wash your hands, use the toilet, and change diapers.

Cover your mouth and nose when coughing and sneezing.

Use tissues to blow and clean the nose, then remove them correctly.

I don't spit.

If you are sick, stay home.

If you still feel bad after treatment with antibiotics, consult your doctor for help.

The number of diseases that receive the title of "superbug" increases over time, but at the moment the following list is relevant:

Staphylococcus aureus - MRSA) - found on the mucous membrane and human skin, MRSA was one of the earlier bacteria in which it was detected resistance to penicillin in 1947. This disease is very common and is responsible for many deaths in the hospital.

Streptococcus and Enterococcus-to eliminate them; you need a combination of antibiotics. Streptococcus is responsible for pneumonia, bacteremia, otitis media, meningitis, sinusitis, peritonitis, and arthritis.

Pseudomonas aeruginosa-this is a widespread opportunistic pathogen. It has a low sensitivity to antibiotics.

Clostridium nosocomial pathogen that causes diarrhea diseases in hospitals around the world. Some studies suggest that Clostridium

Colitis is caused by excessive use of antibiotics in livestock.

Salmonella and E. coli-these are often the result of drinking contaminated water. They became more dangerous, with more deaths, due to the widespread use of antibiotics.

Acineto bacter Baumannii-5. November 2004, the Center for Disease Control and Prevention (CDC) reported that a growing number of people who suffer from Acineto bacter has in the medical devices or soldiers who have fought in Iraq or Kuwait.

Klebsiella Pneumoniae-an emerging gram-negative Bacillus highly resistant to medications, which cause infections associated with significant morbidity and mortality, with a rapidly increasing incidence in a variety of clinical settings around the world.

Mycobacterium Tuberculosis-multidrug-resistant tuberculosis is responsible for 150,000 deaths per year. An increase in the HIV / AIDS epidemic contributed to this. Tuberculosis was considered one of the most widespread diseases and had no treatment until Selman Waksman discovered streptomycin in 1943. However, bacteria soon, resistance has evolved. Since then, drugs such as isoniazid and rifampicin have been used. Mycobacterium Tuberculosis develops drug Resistance through spontaneous mutations in its genomes.

Neisseria Gonorrhoeae is a sexually transmitted pathogen that can cause pelvic pain, pain during urination, penis and vaginal discharge, as well as systemic symptoms in human infection. Records of the bacterium indicate that it was first identified in 1879. Treatment with penicillin was effective at 40. years, but at 70over the years, a drug-resistant strain has evolved.

These superbugs often need to be treated with a combination of powerful antibiotics. Experts and scientists are constantly trying to find the weakness of these viruses to give them a convenient opportunity to fight them.

Here is the important quote from one of the scientists who have dedicated their work to this "discovery of a fungus capable of rendering these multidrug-resistant organisms incapable of further infection is huge," says Irena Kenneley, a microbiologist and infectious disease specialist at Frances Payne Bolton School of Nursing at Case Western Reserve University in Cleveland. "The availability of more treatment options will ultimately save many more lives."

Because the use of antibiotics in agriculture (which promotes the growth and prevents infection in animals) contributed to the mutation of resistant infections, one way to give more chance there is to consume only meat that has been reared on organic farms.

There are other, more natural means that you can use to help your immune system fight these bacteria, and include:

Tea tree oil has a proven ability to fight and kill staphylococcal bacteria. It is used as a topical application, going directly to the infected skin.

Apple cider vinegar and baking soda-a mixture of these two components, you can make a paste that works similar to tea tree oil.

Garlic-a complex composition of garlic is ideal for stimulating the immune system and fighting infections.

Coriander oil - a study conducted in 2011 by Portuguese researchers found that coriander oil is effective against 12 lethal bacteria.

Pascalite-this is a kind of bentonite clay, which is found only in the Wyoming mountains. With local use, its ability to attract wound infections is known within a few hours or days, which leads to complete recovery.

Turmeric-a medicinal product that has been used for centuries to combat bacterial and viral infections. Proven anti-inflammatory and antibacterial properties.

Honey Makuna-in combination with turmeric provides a powerful remedy for the treatment of MRSA and other superbugs.

Oregano oil-has a proven ability to fight bacteria and staphylococcal infections.

Extract of olive leaf-contains the active compound, which provides support to the immune system in the fight against infections resistant to antibiotics.

Echinacea-it is mainly used today to combat colds and flu, but it is traditionally used to treat open wounds, diphtheria, cellulites, blood poisoning, syphilitic lesions, and other bacterial diseases. It contains the ability to destroy even the most demanding bacteria.

Colloidal silver-germicides and antibacterial properties of colloidal silver were discovered almost a century. Numerous clinical cases and anecdotal evidence allow us to know that colloidal silver can kill bacteria, fungal infections, and viruses.

Pau d'arco - which is a plant native to South America whose active ingredient order has been found to relieve a wide range of infections, including those initiated by bacteria, viruses, and fungi.

So, as you can see, although there are currently no known treatments for these superbugs, there are things that we can do to protect yourself and help in the fight against these bacteria, with traditional and herbal medicines.

The Use of Antibiotics-Everything You Need to Know

The choice of taking herbal antibiotics is very personal. As noted in the last chapter, all information is the key to changing the way of life when taking herbal medicines-including antibiotics. You need to make sure that they are suitable for you. Of course, in emergency situations such as acute illness or trauma, this can lead to the work of traditional antibiotics. That herbal medicines work best is prevention, chronic diseases, and the subsequent effects left by these antibiotics.

The study presented here shows that almost a third of Americans use herbal remedies. Although there are things you can consider to make sure that they are suitable for you and your health:

Other medicines you are taking - you will need to see your doctor to make sure that they do not behave badly.

Side effects - although herbal remedies have much fewer options side effects compared to conventional antibiotics, you should always know what options are if they assign.

Regulation-herbal remedies are not regulated as a joint treatment. There are many resources and information that will help you make a decision, but some groups have not been adequately tested on pregnant or nursing women, children, or the elderly.

Infection can be described in two parts heat and moisture." This suggests that antibiotics are excellent for the treatment of "heat" is part of the infection-fever, sore throat, inflammation-due to the fact that often leave the symptoms of "wet" – mucus, nausea, foggy head-the only one. Therefore, many herbalists often recommend herbal treatment with conventional medicine.

Antibiotics are mainly used for bacterial infections, such as:

Conditions that are not particularly severe, but are unlikely to be clarified without the use of antibiotics, such as moderate acne.

Conditions that are not especially serious but could spread to other people if not promptly treated, such as the skin infection impetigo or the sexually transmitted infection Chlamydia.

Conditions where evidence suggests that antibiotics could significantly accelerate recovery, such as kidney infection.

Conditions that carry the risk of more serious complications, such as cellulite or pneumonia.

The formation of antibiotics began in 1877 when Louis Pasteur found that the growth of the coal of the bacteria responsible for the disease could be inhibited by saprophytic bacteria. Then, in 1928, the most important contribution to the world of antibiotics was when Alexander Flemming made a discovery that led to penicillin. Since the ' 70s. For years, most of the new antibiotics were synthetic modifications of antibiotics present in nature.

The process of the formation of antibiotics is fermentation. If you are interested in this process, the steps are as follows:

1. Before the beginning of fermentation, the organism that produces the necessary antibiotics should be isolated, and its number should be increased several times. For this, a starter culture is formed in the laboratory from a sample of previously isolated and cold organisms. When cultivating the initial culture, the sample of the organism is transferred to a plate containing Agar. The initial culture is then put in bottles of a mixture with food and other

nutrients necessary for growth. This creates a suspension, which can be transferred to growth reservoirs.

2. Seed tanks are steel tanks designed to provide an ideal environment for the growth of microorganisms. They are full of all the things a specific microorganism would need to survive and prosper, including hot water foods and carbohydrates such as lactose or glucose sugar. In addition, they contain other necessary carbon sources such as acetic acid, alcohols or hydrocarbons, and the sources of nitrogen, such as ammonia salts. Growth factors such as vitamins, amino acids, and small nutrients surround the composition of the seeds of the contents of the tray. Tank seeds are equipped with mixers, which keep the growing medium moving and a pump, which ensure a sterilized and filtered air. After about 24-28 hours, the material in the tanks is transferred to the primary tanks for fermentation.

3. The fermentation tank is essentially a larger version of the steel tank with seeds, which is able to hold about 30,000 gallons. It is filled with the same growth medium, located in a seed tank, and also provides an inductive growth environment. Here microorganisms can grow and multiply. During this process, they secrete a large amount

of the desired antibiotic. The tanks shall be cooled to maintain a temperature between 23 and 27 ° f (73 and 81 ° F). 2 ° C). Constantly stirring, a constant stream of sterilized air flows out. For this reason, anti-foaming agents are regularly added. Since pH control is necessary for optimal growth, they are added to the reservoir with the necessary acid or base.

4. After three to five days, the maximum amount of antibiotics is formed, and the process of isolation can begin. Depending on the antibiotic produced, the fermentation broth is treated with various cleaning methods. For example, for water-soluble antibiotic compounds, ion exchange method can be used for purification. In this process, the compound is separated from the organic waste in the broth and sent to the device that separates other compounds needed water-soluble compounds. To isolate an oil-soluble antibiotic, such as penicillin, a solvent extraction method is used. In this method, the broth is treated with organic solvents, such as butyl acetateor methylisobutyl ketone, which can specifically dissolve the antibiotic. The dissolved antibiotic is then obtained with the help of various organic chemical means. At the end of this phase, manufacturers usually

leave a purified powder form of the antibiotic, which can be refined into different types of products.

5. Antibiotics can take many different forms. It can be sold in solutions for intravenous bags or syringes in a pill or gel capsule or can be sold in powder form, which is incorporated into topical ointments. Depending on the final form of the antibiotic, several stages of refining can be taken after the initial isolation. Crystalline antibiotics can be dissolved in the solution for intravenous bags, put in a bag, which is then firmly closed. With gel capsules is the antibiotic pill, which physically fills the bottom half of the capsule, and the upper half is placed mechanically. When used in local ointments, the antibiotic is mixed in the ointment.

6. Now the antibiotic is transported to the last packing station. Here the products are stored and placed in boxes. They are loaded on trucks and transported to various distributors, hospitals, and pharmacies. The whole process of fermentation, recovery, and treatment can last from five to eight days.

This antibiotic acts by the difference between the structure of bacterial cells and the host cell. They prevent the multiplication of bacterial cells, leaving their number the same, allowing the body to fight with natural defense or completely kill bacteria.

These antibiotics can be administered in one of three ways:

Orally-tablets, pills, and capsules or a liquid that you drink, which can be used to treat most types of mild to moderately severe infections in the body.

Topical-creams, creams, sprays, or drops, which are often used to treat skin infections.

Injections - these injections can be administered as injections or drip infusions directly into the blood or into the muscle and are usually reserved for more serious infections.

Synthetic antibiotics can be divided into six different categories:

Penicillins are widely used to treat various infections, including skin infections, chest infections, and urinary tract infections.

Cephalosporins can be used to treat a wide range of infections but are also effective in treating more serious infections, such as septicemia and meningitis.

Aminoglycosides are used only to treat very serious diseases, such as sepsis, because they can cause serious side effects, including hearing loss and kidney damage. They quickly break inside the digestive system, so they need to be injected. They are also used as drops for some ear or eye infections.

Tetracyclines can be used to treat a wide range of infections. They are commonly used to treat moderate to severe acne, and a condition called rosacea, which causes redness of the skin and spots.

Macrolides can be especially useful in the treatment of pulmonary and thoracic infections. They can also be a useful alternative for people with allergies to penicillin or to treat strains of penicillin-resistant bacteria.

Fluoroquinolones are broad-spectrum antibiotics that can be used to treat a wide range of infections.

But what were natural antibiotics? How do you decide which ones are right for you? No, there are plenty of places where you can get information about a doctor or pharmacist being one of these sources. Of course, you can try to encourage you to stick with traditional medication, but if you stick to your guns, they will be very useful in what it can and cannot accept, because of the current medication list. Of course, to decide whether herbal medicines for you are right as soon as I couldn't find anywhere that they are safe for you to take - the best thing you can do is try. Once you have tried the recommended dose, you will know how effective it is for your body.

In many cases, scientists aren't sure which specific ingredient in a particular herb works to treat disease or illness. Whole herbs contain many ingredients and can work together to have a beneficial effect. Efficacy has been determined by many factors. For example, the type of environment (climate, bugs, soil quality) in which the plant will have an impact on how and when it WAS collected and processed.

Natural antibiotics work in two ways, eliminate dangerous bacteria and strengthen the natural defenses of the body. There are many foods, was and spices that have the necessary natural antibiotic properties.

Some Examples With Information on How They Work-are Listed Below:

Oregano Oil

There are many components and foods that naturally have antibiotic activity. For example, oregano oil contains a high concentration of thymol and carvacrol, two strong antibacterial and antifungal compounds. They can help prevent secondary bacterial infections. Oregano essential oil is very effective against a number of microorganisms in Tests against other antimicrobial oils. Studies show that it is an effective antibiotic against Staphylococcus aureus (staphylococcus))

Oregano oil may be useful in the treatment of respiratory tract infections, gastrointestinal disorders, menstrual cramps, and urinary TRACT infections. It can also be applied locally to skin conditions to control acne or dandruff.

Honey

Honey, as food has a natural anti-inflammatory activity, but not all honey is formed in the same way. Manuka honey from New Zealand contains other goods such as methylglyoxal (MG). It is believed that MG gives antibacterial properties to Manuka honey. Manuka is best for wound treatment. However, it is a honey medic that is sterilized and packaged as a wound bandage.

Garlic

Garlic has a long history of use as an antibacterial agent. Due to the lack of penicillin in the Second World War, canceled doctors turned to Czechoslovakia. "Today, with an increase in antibiotic-resistant bacteria, there is a renewed interest in the study, the active substance of garlic. Allicin breaks down in the heat, so it must be swallowed raw. Crude Czech oil can also be effective as a local antimicrobial,"

Says McCrae. The uses include treatment of colds and flu, fungal infections, warts, hypertension, and garlic may have potential in serious disorders, such as diabetes, heart disease, and some cancers.

Tea Tree Oil

Tea tree oil is antiseptic and effective against some strains of bacteria. It has been proved that the oil of the Melaleuca tree species is the most effective and least irritating to the skin. Tea tree oil is used in skin diseases such as acne, fungal infections, and athlete's foot, as well as a vaginal infection, herpes on the mouth or ear infections.

Elderberry Happy

Series of recent studies stress the immune-strengthening effect of elderberry water-based extracts and juice, as well as free radicals scavenging activity, which is able to protect cells from damage, infection, and disease. In the fight against influenza, cough, colds, and intent, almonds, blue, or blackberries were used. Their antioxidant benefits can also play a role in lowering bad cholesterol and some cancers.

Berberine

Nopal occurs in the berberine, which occurs naturally In several herbs, such as barberry (Berberi Vulgaris), has a broad spectrum of antibiotic activity on a long history of medicinal use In Chinese and Ayurvedic medicine. Berberine exhibits antimicrobial activity against bacteria, viruses, fungi, protozoa, and worms. It is widely used for the prevention of many types of infections, especially eye infections and bacterial diarrhea. In recent studies, Berberine and goldenseal extract are strongly inhibited by influenza.

Andrographis

Andrograph is a herbal stimulant the most reliable on the basis of several human clinical trials against upper respiratory infections, to reduce the severity of the symptoms (in particular pain in the neck), as well as expectoration, nasal secretion, headache, fever, pain fish soup, malaise/fatigue, and sleep disorders.

A multicenter study, including John Hopkins, found " herbal therapies are at least as effective as Rifaximin with a "similar response rate and safety profiles." A previous study, Dr. Logan, used to enter solvent mint oil (ECPO) in a patient with mild results. This is just one of many studies that show how effective the drugs are.

You can see for yourself the following video about antibiotics vs. botanical therapies and supplements

Were drugs are also great for dealing with side effects left by antibiotics.

They may include the following list:

Chronic sinus congestion

Fatigue, heaviness or fog

Recurrent infections of the sinuses or bladder

The urgency of urination or pressure

Chronic yeast infection

Loose stool, swelling or loss of appetite

Nausea or nausea

Abdominal pain or diarrhea

Here are some complementary procedures to take care of your body while using antibiotics:

Probiotics-restore good bacteria of the body.

Herbal tea against nausea.

Milk Thistle-on the antioxidant effect on the liver.

You should:

Eat onions and Czech to support the liver and keep the yeast in check.

With omega 3, vitamin C and E and Oregon grape root.

Make sure you consume a well-balanced diet.

Of course, there are pros and cons to both antibiotics and more natural remedies.

These facts should be taken into account when deciding what to take.

Benefits of antibiotics

These are some of the most significant advantages of taking antibiotics:

Can treat many infections: antibiotics can treat a variety of infections, such as sore throat, tonsillitis, and sinusitis.

Easy to inject: most antibiotics are easy to inject because I can inject orally or by injection.

There are several side effects: many antibiotics have few side effects, which makes them the perfect choice when you feel very bad.

Cost effectiveness: most of the older types of antibiotics- especially those with generic alternatives-are often very affordable for every budget, even if you lack health insurance.

Disadvantages of antibiotics

Although there are many advantages of antibiotics, there are also several disadvantages, such as:

Allergic reactions: depending on your allergy medication, you can be very allergic to some types of antibiotics, such as those that contain sulfonamides. Unfortunately, sulfur is present In many common antibiotics, so it may be more difficult to find a suitable cure for your disease.

Resistant bacteria: if you do not take the entire dose of antibiotics to just kill some of the bacteria in the system and can Rest resistant to antibiotics, which means that antibiotics may not work for you in the future.

Potential side effects: while many antibiotics have various side effects, some may cause problems such as unpleasant digestive problems, discomfort, nausea, diarrhea, and sensitivity to light.

In addition, a Finnish study shows that the effects of antibiotics on intestinal bacteria were still visible after a year. That is, the following effects of taking antibiotics are harmful for a long time. Constant overuse of antibiotics will lead to the formation of resistant bacteria and further unnecessary death; therefore, if possible, we should use herbal antibiotic therapy.

Benefits of natural remedies

There are a number of advantages associated with the use of herbal medicines, unlike pharmaceutical preparations:

Reduced risk of side effects: most herbal drugs are well-tolerated patients, with fewer undesirable consequences than medications. Herbs usually have fewer side effects than traditional medicine and can be safer to use over time.

Effective with chronic diseases: herbal medicines tend to be more effective for long-term health problems that do not respond well to traditional medicine. An example of these are herbs and drugs used to treat arthritis. Vioxx, a well-known prescription drug used to treat arthritis, has been remembered because of the increased risk of cardiovascular complications. Alternative treatments for arthritis, on the other hand, have several side effects. Such treatments include changes in diet, such as adding simple herbs, eliminating vegetables from the nightshade family, and reducing the consumption of white sugar.

Lower cost: another advantage of Phytotherapy is the price. Herbs cost much less than prescription drugs. Research, testing, and marketing contribute significantly to the cost of prescription drugs. Herbs tend to be cheap compared to drugs.

Widespread availability: another advantage of herbal medicines is their availability. Herbs are available without a prescription. You can grow simple herbs, such as mint and chamomile, at home. In some remote parts of the world, herbs may be the only treatment available to most people.

Disadvantages of natural remedies

Herbs are not without drawbacks, and Phytotherapy is not suitable in all situations. These are some disadvantages that need to be taken into account:

Inappropriate for many conditions: modern medicine treats sudden and serious illnesses and accidents much more effectively than herbal or alternative treatments. An herbalist would not be able to treat a severe trauma, such as a broken leg, nor would it be able to heal appendicitis or a heart attack as efficiently as a conventional doctor using modern diagnostic tests, surgery, and medicines.

The absence of dosage instructions: another drawback of Phytotherapy is a very real risk of harm from self-dosing with herbs. Although it can be argued that the same can happen with medications, such as accidental overdose in the cold, many herbs are not provided with instructions or packaging inserts. There is a very real risk of overdose.

Poison risk associated with wild herbs: harvesting herbs in nature is risky, if not risky, but some people try to identify and collect wild herbs. They would risk poisoning if they did not correctly identify the grass or using the wrong part of the plant.

Drug interactions: herbal treatments can interact with drugs. Nearly all herbs come with a warning, and many, like the herbs used for anxiety such as valerian and St. John's wort, can interact with prescription drugs such as antidepressants. It is important to discuss herbal medicines and supplements with your doctor to avoid dangerous interactions.

Lack of regulation: because plant products are not strictly regulated, consumers are also at risk of buying substandard herbs. The quality of plant products may vary by batch, brand, or manufacturer. This can make it much more difficult to prescribe the right dose of grass.

From these lists, it is obvious why they are herbal antibiotics used for centuries – for a long time, compared to what was created by synthetic antibiotics. I work.

With our body fighting bacteria and infections, that's why we have far fewer side effects left. Even when it is necessary to take antibiotics by prescription, herbal medicines are great for maintaining a healthy body and fighting all the side effects that may occur.

BREAKING THE ANTIBIOTIC CYCLE

You have a sinus infection or a bladder infection; ask for medical treatment, and you are prescribed an antibiotic; after stopping the antibiotic, do your symptoms return after seeing the doctor for other antibiotics? Before you know it, your symptoms do not disappear and always take several antibiotics for longer and longer periods.

Or maybe you take an antibiotic every day to try to keep the symptoms of infection at bay?

Unfortunately, you're not alone. Antibiotics are the first class of prescription drugs in the United States, with about 84 million written prescriptions written each year during office visits and 40 million prescriptions after discharge from the hospital (CDC, The Hague). It is also estimated by the Centers for Disease Control that only 10% of these antibiotic prescriptions are guaranteed.

The three main causes of infection...

Not all infections are similar, although they seem to cause the same general symptoms: pain, swelling, redness, discharge, fever, pain, and general fatigue. However, the agents that cause infection are different:

Virus. Viruses are small pieces of genetic code that enter a sensitive cell and assume its functions, saying that the cell to make more of the virus. The immune system quickly destroys viruses once detected. Viruses "their term" which means that each virus has a habitual delay in which it causes signs of the disease before the immune system destroys. Viruses account for almost 75% of all ear, sinus, and upper respiratory tract infections.

Mushroom. Fungi are a type of mold. Inside the body of everyone (in the ears, nose, vagina, bladder, intestines, and intestines), there is a special kind of fungus. It's Candida albicans. This fungus must be present to protect the body and help the intestines break down food. When there is too much Candida, it can produce signs of infection.

The Mayo Clinic estimates that Candida infections account for 98% of all recurrent infections and about 15% of new infections.

Bacterial. Bacteria are cells in themselves. When they enter a sensitive area of the body, they multiply and produce more bacterial cells. A healthy immune system can destroy bacteria; if the immune system is not strong enough, a bacterial infection can continue. Bacterial infections account for about 10% of all infections.

Parasite. These are listed because parasitic infections can occur. Most often, this kind of infection occurs from uncooked pork products. Some scientists believe that everyone on the planet has a parasitic infection and contributed to many health problems to parasites. However, many people do not have signs of infection with parasites. Less than 1% of infections are the result of parasites.

How Antibiotics Work

There are 17 different classes of antibiotics; however, each class works similarly. Each antibiotic is a general ("broad spectrum") or specific ("concentrated") antibiotic. A broad-spectrum antibiotic is designed to eliminate a variety of similar bacteria. A targeted antibiotic targets only one or two specific bacteria. If you did not receive a test before being prescribed an antibiotic, you would have received a broad-spectrum antibiotic; almost all prescribed antibiotics are broad-spectrum.

Note that antibiotics affect bacteria. Bacteria are cells in themselves. Our body consists of many cells. Cells are individual units in the body that are separated from other cells by a shell, so to speak. The shells of bacteria are different from the shells of the cells of our body. Thus, the immune system can search and identify what is not part of the body.

An antibiotic can do the same. When a person takes an antibiotic, he looks for shells that have a certain identifier; then, he destroys these cells cutting a hole in the shell of bacteria. The cell dies, so the bacteria die.

Unfortunately, broad-spectrum antibiotics do not know the difference between good bacteria and those that cause infection. Our bodies contain bacteria necessary for the digestion of food, the absorption of vitamins and minerals, and the nutrient mucosa. When an antibiotic works, it will also destroy these bacteria.

(It should be noted that special "antibiotics" are for parasitic infections (such as Actelion), viral infections (such as Tamiflu), and fungal infections (such as Mycostatin or Lamisil). These are not those discussed in this article, as these are rarely prescribed and are not those prescribed abundantly.)

For other causes of infection?

Since antibiotics only work on bacteria, they will not work on viruses, fungal infections, or parasites. If you take an antibiotic for an infection caused by a virus, parasite, or fungus, the infection will not improve.

But I feel better when I take an antibiotic.

The signs of an infection are actually signs that the immune system is fighting the infection. When an antibiotic is taken, the body's healing efforts are stopped because a new, more toxic substance has entered the body. Infection is harmful (that's why your body was fighting it), but toxic chemicals are more harmful, so dealing with them has priority for the health of the body. Even if the infection is caused by a virus, the symptoms of such an infection will decrease or disappear because the body has something more harmful to focus on. Remember: the signs of an infection are the immune system that fights infection. Without the immune system that fights infection, the symptoms will decrease or disappear until the drug disappears or is "managed" by the body.

Is repeated (chronic) use of antibiotics safe?

Not counting allergic reactions to antibiotics, there are many documented cases of adverse reactions; the most common is diarrhea and nausea. In the digestive system (intestines and stomach) are good bacteria that help digestion and assimilation of nutrients. When these good bacteria are killed by the antibiotic, digestion is disrupted, and the good yeast (Candida albicans) that exists in the intestine has more room to grow, so it is. Remember, yeast is not killed by antibiotics. Not only is there an excess of yeast growth, but there may be a decrease in the absorption of nutrients and difficulties in breaking down the consumed food, which leads to diarrhea and the risk of nutritional deficiencies.

Another not often discussed effect is, in fact, immune suppression. As mentioned above, the immune system slows down when the body has to deal with chemical toxins / foreign substances. If a person has a virus, the virus will continue to do more than itself, unhindered by an immune system. Once the antibiotic is stopped, the virus will show itself again, but it will be stronger because it had the opportunity to take a stronger take. In addition, the fungal infection discussed in the previous paragraph will worsen during the antibiotic; it was also not hampered by an immune system. With yeast throughout the body, it is possible that the signs of recurrent infection in the sinuses or bladder, for example, are caused by yeast. As mentioned above, the Mayo Clinic estimates that 98% of recurrent infections are the result of yeast, not bacteria, so recurrent antibiotics in these cases would not have helped the situation.

Chronic fatigue syndrome has been associated with chronic infections, as a result of scarring responses weakened by chronic antibiotic use.

A new concern that has arisen concerns autoimmune disorders. It has been suggested and is now being studied that taking stimulating supplements while taking antibiotics increases the risk of a person developing an auto-immune disorder because the immune system is confused when it is suppressed and stimulated at the same time.

Another problem with the chronic use of antibiotics (will not be discussed here, however) is the development of "superbugs," bacteria that cannot be destroyed by antibiotics typical because (the bacteria) had been exposed to antibiotics so often that they are now "immune" against them.

How can the cycle be broken?

The immune system is designed to search for and neutralize any invader, whether bacterial, viral, parasitic, fungal, or otherwise. The stronger the immune system, the faster the response to these foreign invaders will be.

What can I do?

Remember that diseases do not occur in a vacuum, which means that there is no reason why a disease affects and why it can stay around. Always consider the emotions that are aroused by the disease or the emotions that may have started the problems. Each area of the body contains stronger emotions than others; for example, the bladder is afraid; the nose, sadness, and despair.

Also, look at your living and working environments. If you have a chronic sinus infection, do you live in a house that has mold? Do you work in an area that has been painted fresh? Look at your personal habits. Do you often hold the bladder so that you go to the toilet only twice a day? Smoke?

It is also a good idea to supplement your diet with probiotics, such as acidophilus. With antibiotics that destroy good bacteria in the body, these good bacteria need to be replaced. There are many acidophilic or probiotic formulas on the market, or eat one yogurt a day, the one that has "live yogurt crops."

You Know What?

If you want to break the antibiotic cycle and stop suffering, know that it can be done! You have the symptoms of an infection because your body is fighting to get rid of it, which means all you have to do is give it a little help, and the body will do the rest. You do not have to suffer the rest of your days; you do not have to put your life, creativity, and joy because of a chronic infection. Know that there are options. Know that you can be free from your sufferings.

HERBAL REMEDIES TO PREVENT ANTIBIOTIC CAUSED SERIOUS ILLNESSES

There are many definitions of the word madness. One of them is that a person can not understand the nature and consequences of his actions. Another is that the person is a danger to himself or others. Another is that the person dresses in a white dress and goes running on the street shouting "help, the world is on fire."

People think that if they take a herb, a plant, and not a prescription drug, the herbal remedy is not powerful. According to many, herbal remedies were created by God, and drugs were created by mortals. Who is the most powerful? If you do not understand that herbs can be very powerful, then a hemlock salad. Then take two aspirin and call me in the morning.

When antibiotics were discovered, they were called the biggest step forward by the invention of the mp3 player. They were hailed as Caesar. Salad. Antibiotics killed a part of us, bacteria, and kept many alive who would otherwise have died. That is why in the last two thousand years the population of the Earth has increased from 1 million to 6 billion. It should reach 9 billion by 2050 when we have eaten all the herbs and will be forced to live exclusively on artificial food. When Karl Benz invented the car 150 years ago, it was thought to be the biggest discovery since Lana Turner at the soda stand. Without cars, today we would not invade the Middle East for their oil, and greenhouse gases would not melt the Arctic and Antarctica. The ocean wouldn't have increased by 50 feet, and Kevin Costner wouldn't have blown up a package on Waterworld. Who knew?

The bad news is that antibiotics have horrible side effects. Imagine that your body is a large salad bowl. Take my salad bowl. Please. Inside this salad bowl, there are white flakes, your healthy bacteria, your flora and fauna, and Black weeds, unhealthy bacteria, toxic germs. When the antibiotic happens in the belly, colon, and bloodstream, it kills germs. The bad news is that it also kills healthy bacteria, white flakes. Once you finish taking antibiotics for a week, only black weeds, mushrooms, yeast remain in your salad bowl. These yeast fungi are live animals that then begin to have their own population explosion. Soon they have taken control of your colon and begin to eat their way through the colon into the bloodstream, which then takes in every cell of your body. The Candida yeast then begins to coat and eat through your organs until you develop all the diseases in the book. An ounce of prevention is worth a pound of healing, especially when there is no cure.

You may begin to develop depression, fatigue, yeast infections, emphysema, which is where the lungs look like Swiss cheese, and you sit in agony in a wheelchair with a mask attached to the oxygen cylinders. You're welcome, Dr. Frankenstein. You can't believe your doctor would do this to you. If not, ask why doctors distribute Paxil to suicidal patients when they are fully aware that Paxil makes the patient more likely to commit suicide. Or you can ask why your inbox is full of Viagra ads when your doctor knows very well that Viagra causes blindness. The list of side effects of prescription drugs that cause short- and long-term death is endless. It's about money. That is why Jesus overthrew the tables of money changers and called the Holy Temple a den of Thieves. Your local pharmacy is not a sacred temple. It can not even be located in Jerusalem.

Sometimes antibiotics are great for killing bacteria that are going to kill you. If you need to take them, after you finish, start taking acidophilus. Acidophilus capsules contain billions of healthy bacteria. These healthy bacteria are also found in yogurt. These herbal remedies, flora, and fauna begin to multiply and fill your salad bowl with healthy white flakes and leave the black weeds nowhere to grow. Also, take grapefruit seed extract pills that kill black weeds. The most important is to take oregano.

The most powerful antibiotic in nature is oregano. The oregano Herbal Remedy has been clinically proven to kill bacteria that the strongest antibiotic cannot, viruses, mold, fungi, yeast, and black weeds in your salad bowl. The herbal remedy oregano is available in several forms. It is sold in your store of natural foods such as oregano oil and oregano capsules. You can use the dropper to put directly under the tongue or in a little grapefruit juice. The good thing about oregano is that it does not kill white flakes. Instead, it promotes their growth as it kills Black weeds.

Many people suffer from sinusitis. Sinusitis is often just a bunch of molds that is naturally in the air we breathe, and bacteria, fungi, and parasites in the cavities of the sinus. Oregano often kills them and heals sinusitis. Many children and adults suffer from allergies. Often it is simply airborne mold that reproduces in the lungs. Oregano enters the bloodstream with sage and cumin, other herbal remedies in the same capsule, and kills the mold that reproduces in the lungs, eradicating the cause of Allergy and ending asthma, bronchitis, and emphysema.

Millions of people are caught in a vicious circle. A drug leads to new diseases that require new drugs that cause new diseases that require new drugs until you are standing at the pharmacy counter with a bag full of pills in terrible suffocating pain until death. The reason that large pharmaceutical companies do not advertise oregano is that it grows in nature, they cannot patent it and cannot get money from it. This does not mean that you should not run to your health food store immediately or online and buy these herbal remedies and kill your toxic black weeds and start cultivating your flora and fauna.

THE IMMUNE SYSTEM

The immune system is a buzzing machine of complexity. It maintains the basic ability to remember past illnesses and prevent the body from returning to stress and illness. In addition, it has an improved communication system that provides the necessary response to the reaction caused by an infection or wound. Immune cells create the right secretions, which further strengthen the "fighting" immune cells. However, the body's immune system may weaken, resulting in gout disease. It works on stronger immunity by eating well, resting well, exercising, being in the sun, and reducing stress levels.

As has been said, synthetic antibiotics can effectively hinder the immune system, refuting good bacteria in places and allows the growth of harmful bacteria in a weak immune system. Look for the following immunostimulant herbs to maintain the immune system. The immune system is strengthened by supporting the stomach. It is well documented that people suffering from malnutrition worldwide are more at risk of disease. Therefore, it is important to feed well with the following herbs.

GINSENG

Ginseng is found all over the world in different varieties. Panax ginseng, or Korean ginseng, is perhaps the most common. Its main component, ginsenoside, contains anti-inflammatory and antitumor attributes. Supports the immune system and healing cells from any damage to free radicals to the environment or choosing the wrong diet. In addition, it is known that it fights diabetes.

Asian Chicken Soup with Ginseng

Note: This recipe is excellent in repairing and healing the spleen and stomach, as well as strengthening the body's immune system. It uses root fibers, small cords that fall from the main root of the ginseng plant.

Gross:

- Four chicken thighs
- Fivered dates, 10 g of ginseng fiber two slices of ginger root one tsp. salt
- Six cups of water

Instruction:

First, cut the chicken thighs into two pieces. Bring to a boil a saucepan of two cups of water, then cook the chicken in water for thirty seconds. Then remove the chicken from the boiling water and drain the chicken.

On the side, place the chicken, ginseng, dates, ginger root, and water together in a safe, heat-resistant bowl. Spray the ingredients of the dish together in a steamer or in a wok over boiling water. Continue to heat for two hours and constantly restore the water supply as soon as the water evaporates. After two hours, remove the soup from the heat and serve hot.

Ginger

Ginger, root with a hard and ugly exterior, impulses with anti-inflammatory properties. Ginger actually works to eliminate the reaction of certain genes that cause inflammation. Inflammation is perhaps the number one killer, the main cause of all diseases of the body, such as cancer, diabetes, and colds. Since cellular inflammation is reduced, it actively refutes future disease. In addition, ginger acts in the fight against blood clots, hypercholesterolemia, and cardiovascular diseases.

Tuna Tartare With Ginger Pepper

Folder:

Two onions

One lb. tuna

1-inch ginger root

Onered pepper

Six tbsp. soy sauce

One tbsp. honey

Two tbsp. sesame oil juice of 1 lime

Four slices of bread:

Start with the preparation of tuna. We cut the tuna into cubes, remove all the dark parts of the bloody line. Put the tuna in a large bowl and leave the fish fresh.

Prepare the vegetables: chopped red pepper, onion, and ginger root. Add the onions, chili, and ginger to the tuna bowl and mix.

On the side, mix soy sauce, lime juice, honey, and sesame oil.

Also, pour this mixture with tuna and continue to stir.

Grill each piece of bread in a toaster or on a plate. Serve tartar on toast, or directly on the side of toast, for a delicious experience.

Turmeric

Turmeric is an ancient Indian herb that contains curcumin. Curcumin is rich in antioxidants that refute inflammation caused by free radicals in the body. In addition, it calms the stomach by increasing the flow of bile and against bacterial infections. Turmeric stimulates the adrenal glands in the body in order to increase the hormone, which reduces the signs of internal inflammation. Other studies show that turmeric better protects the liver, so it may be a toxin derived from the high consumption of the alcohol contained with the use of turmeric.

Ginger and turmeric tea

It eliminates internal pain and increases the immune system with the rejuvenating properties of turmeric and ginger.

Folder:

¼ Tsp.z.From. Ground turmeric ¼ tsp. ginger

1 tbsp. soy milk

1 tsp. z. From. honey

Direction:

Start by boiling water from the Cup in a bowl. Pour turmeric and ginger and reduce to low heat. Let the water and ingredients boil for about ten minutes. So pour in the milk and mix well. Lubricate the mixture into a cup of tea and add honey for sweets.

Turmeric of the Western Wonder

Folder:

1 tbsp. oil

14 to 16 ounces tofu

½ Cup red pepper ¼ cup white onion ¼ teaspoon. coriander

½ Cup Anaheim Pepper ¼ tsp. Garlic powder ¼ tsp. cumin

1 ½ tsp. z. From. turmeric

½ Tsp. z. From. Salt

Direction:

First, remove the tofu from the package and put it on a dry cloth. Dry with paper towels until more water is removed. Then put it in a bowl and use a fork to crush it. Tofu should fall apart.

On the side, heat the olive oil in a medium-fried frying pan. When heated for a while, prepare chili, white onion, and Anaheim pepper by cutting and cutting into cubes. Throw them in the oil. Cook for four minutes, stirring occasionally.

Then add cumin, coriander, garlic powder, and salt to the pepper-onion mixture and continue stirring for one minute. Add crushed tofu and turmeric. Cook for about two more minutes and season with salt and pepper, if desired. This recipe can be eaten alone or served in warmed tortillas with avocado accompaniments.

Ganoderma

This Asian herb is a bitter mushroom. It is used in Chinese medical practice of several centuries, and recent studies show that grass increases immunity and fights with the first signs of cancer. It also contains antioxidants that reduce inflammation in the body by providing internal relief. Take a look at this herb, especially if you hope to reduce pain from urinary tract infections. The best way to use Ganoderma for its healthy properties is to drink tea with reishi mushrooms.

Reishi Mushroom Tea

Folder:

Five grams of dried mushrooms reishi (try the brand Mountain Rose Herb from the local grocery store)

Three cups of water

Direction:

Breakage ganoderma is incredibly difficult; many argue that during the process of breaking coffee grinders or food processors. Use what you have. Try a heavy blade or carefully, fingers. Or buy a ready-made bag from reishi.

Bring three cups of water to a boil. Add pieces of mushrooms to boiling water and reduce the temperature of the hob to a low level. Let the water boil for two hours.

So, strain the water and put the tea on the side. Let the tea cool down for a couple of minutes before drinking it. Note: tea is stored for up to three days in the refrigerator.

Cat Claw

The common use of Peruvian grass, a cat's claw, is to treat stomach problems. However, it has been shown that recent use increases the immune system. It stimulates the immune system, allows the secretion of a greater number of cells to fight. In addition, the cat's claw contains oxindole alkaloids, which increases the body's ability to ingest and remove bacteria and viruses.

Antiviral Tea That Increases Immunity

Note: this immunity-enhancing tea also contains chuchuhuasi, which is known to reduce joint pain in people.

Gross:

1 tsp. of vanilla

2 tbsp. Goji Berries

½ Tsp. of Bercampuri

1 tbsp. cat claw

1 ½ tbsp chuchuhuasi

Instruction:

First, boil two liters of water in a saucepan, then put all the ingredients in hot water. Let the water boil for ten minutes on low heat. Then soak the ingredients and serve hot.

Ginkgo Biloba

Annoying free radicals in the body from the external environment or poor nutrition are your last days with the use of herbs ginkgo biloba. Gingko biloba leaves contain bilobalides and ginkgolides, which act to refute these free radicals and reduce inflammation. In addition, it turned out that these properties reduce radiation damage. Recent research shows that the herb neutralizes free radicals, which cause cell death due to radiation; in addition, ginkgo reduces damage to brain cells by about fifty percent.

Ginkgo Herbal Tea

Gross:

1 tsp. of ginkgo biloba dried 1 cup water direction:

First, cook 1 cup of water. When it starts to boil, pour the dried herbs. Put on low heat and boil water for twenty minutes. Then pour the water and leave to cool for a while in a cup of coffee. Drink while it's hot.

Rosemary

The ancient Greeks and Romans have long appreciated the beautiful aroma and evergreen nature of this Mediterranean plant. Plant rosemary stimulates the immune system and increases blood circulation, allowing oxygen to enter the cells of the body faster. The brain is strong, with a basic concentration. In addition, this increase in blood flow improves digestion and reduces the hardness of an asthma attack.

Razzmatazz Roasted Sweet Potatoes with Rosemary

Gross:

Six huge sweet potatoes

½ Cup fresh rosemary leaves ½ cup olive oil

1 tbsp. pepper

1 tbsp. salt

Instruction:

Start by preheating the oven to 325 degrees Fahrenheit. Cut the potatoes lengthwise into fried components. Put the fried quarters on a baking sheet and sprinkle the sweet potatoes with 1/3 cup of olive oil. Then sprinkle the chips with rosemary, salt, and pepper.

Put the baking tray in the oven and turn the chips after ten minutes.

Let the chips cook for another twenty minutes.

Before serving, water the sweet potatoes with the rest of the olive oil.

NATURAL REMEDIES FOR YEAST INFECTION

Candida albicans, also known as candidias is, is one of the most confusing to medical science that affects millions of women and men around the world who suffer many times from this state of unconsciousness. Debilitating symptoms of yeast infections are caused by fungal proliferation, which oscillates in severity and occurs in many diseases. Although some doctors have prescribed antibiotics for this condition, research studies have found that herbs for yeast infections, in most cases, surpass pharmaceutical treatment.

One of the problems is that Candida albicans is not alien to the human body; it is the yeast fungus that normally exists in equilibrium with other microorganisms. When the growth rate of this fungus accelerates out of control, the results include thrush; infections that appear as white spots on the tongue and in the mouth and in the throat, which is painful to chew and swallow.

One of the most common causes of Thrush for adults is the use of antibiotics, which, unfortunately, eliminate not only harmful bacteria but also destroy lactobacilli, which is necessary by the body to keep the fungus Candida albicans under control. The fungus develops on high levels of glucose in saliva; people who smoke, wear dentures, or have diabetics are more at risk of developing oral thrush.

Women taking oral contraceptives are at risk of vaginal yeast infections, and thrush can also occur during pregnancy. Due to its adaptability, it can be easily transmitted from mother to child during childbirth or breastfeeding. And with its wide range of symptoms of yeast infection can go unnoticed in areas of the body, such as joints and intestines.

Candida albicans is also associated with poor diet; the typical American diet rich in refined sugars and acidic foods adversely affects the pH balance in the intestine. Long-term stress accelerates the growth of the fungus. Natural remedies for yeast infections work best in combination with proper nutrition.

Commonly Prescribed Herbs for Candida Albicans

Oregano (Origanum compactum):

Essential oil is used as a natural remedy for yeast infections and has a stimulating and warming effect, which can be used internally or externally. Oregano oil contains carvacrol and thymol, which are responsible for its antimicrobial and antimicrobial effects. Research has shown that carvacrol inhibits the growth of Candida albicans. Oregano is also rich in flavonoids, ursolic and oleanolic acids, vitamin A and vitamin C. for its antimicrobial properties, they have proven effective against E. coli and Staphylococcus.

Black Walnut (Juglans Nigra):

One of the most powerful herbs for yeast infections, black walnut is used as antifungal agents; antiseptics to treat and cure Candida albicans. Oxygen the blood and is used to balance sugar, remove toxins and fats. Black walnut copes with Thrush (oral yeast infection), vaginitis (vaginal yeast infection), jock itch (yeast infection), and parasitic infections.

Black walnut as a yeast herbal infection is used to treat intestinal disorders associated with Candida albicans, including irritable bowel syndrome (IBS), parasitic infections of intestinal and intestinal bacterial infections. It is used for indoor and outdoor applications, contains high levels of tannin, juglandin, and juglansacid. Black walnut green skin contains organic iodine, which has antiseptic properties to combat bacterial infections.

Pau D'arco (Tabebuia):

This Phyto-medicinal herbal remedy for yeast infections is made from the bark of the Lapacho tree. The most active compound, Pau D'arco is lapachol, which prevents the growth of mold, acts as a respiratory poison for microorganisms, disrupting their production of oxygen and energy.

Leaves of Neem (Azadirachta Indica):

Neem tree is used in Ayurvedic medicine for its powerful antibacterial and antifungal properties. It is an extremely bitter herb containing alkaloids Azadirachtin and Nimbin. This herb for yeast infections is an invaluable cleanser for skin and blood and is very effective in normalizing intestinal bacteria. Note: pregnant women should not use this herb.

Thor Sturluson is an amateur biologist and herbalist living in Copenhagen, Denmark.

THE MOST EFFECTIVE HOME REMEDIES FOR URINARY TRACT INFECTION

What are the most effective home remedies for urinary tract infection? Natural treatment works by allowing the body to kill or detect E. coli in the urinary tract. But before discussing these three remedies, you need to know that you need to stop taking antibiotics to treat the infection!

The truth about UTI antibiotics

Antibiotics are abused! Listen to leading researchers and scientists about the use of antibiotics in America.

The doctor and Nutritionist, Dr. McDougal, said: "Today, over-prescription and excessive consumption of psychotropic drugs do much more harm than good in our society. Many times, just a few simple lifestyle changes are needed and not too expensive pills with dangerous side effects. Unfortunately, most doctors do not tell us about simple changes in lifestyle, but I don't think twice about prescribing one or two drugs.

Done! If you are taking antibiotics to treat a urinary tract infection, you have a 25% chance of developing an infection in the next few months. Why?

Antibiotics act on urinary tract infection by killing all the bad and good bacteria in the urinary tract or by allowing bacteria to adhere to their peers in the urinary tract. Unfortunately, most ulcers and E. coli are becoming more resistant to most antibiotics.

And that is why thousands of people are now switching to home remedies against urinary tract infections. Here are some of the most popular remains used to treat E. coli.

Three home remedies for urinary tract infections

1. Many people use a simple remedy, which includes unsweetened cranberry juice. Cranberry juice and tablets have been included in many procedures step by step because the compound in the fruit actually makes the bacteria and E. coli already clinging to the walls of the urinary tract. Many sick people drink at least four glasses of juice a day during an attack.

2. Another good idea would be to strengthen the immune system as quickly as possible. You can do it quite effectively replenishes vitamin C and zinc. These two will significantly increase your immune system to start fighting bacteria and coli. We recommend 3000 mg of vitamin C and at least three tablets of zinc per day. Vitamin C tablets should be administered three times a day for 1000 mg.

3. Most people who successfully cure and prevent future attacks will use a multi-ingredient remedy that includes an herbal supplement. An effective herbal remedy that is recommended to try is alfalfa. Concentrates of Alfalfa juice can improve kidney function, and it turns out that healthy kidney functions are important for rinsing urinary tract infections. Alfalfa will help the body get rid of toxins and increase the flow of urine (and, hopefully, bacteria).

A natural remedy for UTI that works in 12 hours!

It discovers and searches, step by step home remedy for UTI that works in 12 hours flat, please visit our website today. Our medicine is approved by a doctor and costs the price of food!

HERBAL ANTIBIOTICS – NATURAL ALTERNATIVES TO SEASONAL SICKNESSES

If you find yourself with a cold that you can not get rid of, you may be surprised to learn that there are effective natural solutions available at any health food store or pharmacy—knowing that you can save on the cost of visiting the office and a trip to the pharmacy.

Some Herbal Antibiotics:

Olive oil/extract is a good natural plant antibiotic. Follow the instructions on the vial, probably take several times a day.

Colloidal silver, another antimicrobial, also works well with it. When using colloidal money, always buy from a reputable company and never exceed the recommended dose. If this happens correctly, it can be a very effective aid in the fight against many common diseases.

Grapefruit oil/extract is also an antibiotic, but it appears to be slightly thicker than the olive leaf. It is better to hide for bad cockroaches like Streptococcus. But I warn you, you need to mix it with liquid to dilute it, and it tastes terrible. Pinch your nose, drink it quickly and bring orange juice or something with a strong taste to drive it away. * Note: do not confuse with grape seed oil.

Oregano oil/extract is also a good antibiotic, but a little softer than the olive leaf. The author gives it to his children when they are cold and usually goes for a ride.

Duration of the course of antibiotics:

Once you start taking antibiotics, I'm sure you're taking 10-14 days, even if you start feeling better earlier just to be sure that the bug comes back. If you have completed the course of antibiotics, but still not better, then do not start again right away, either go to another or look for another method of treatment.

"Friendly Bacteria"

Monitor all antibiotics; of course, whether they are plant, we recommend replenishing "friendly" bacteria by adding things like yogurt (with live crops), sauerkraut, or kimchi to your diet. In addition, you can do this simply in "probiotics" which is in tablet form in some health food stores (look in the fridge). Leaving the "good bacteria" after antibiotic treatment can cause seemingly unrelated, but still bad yeast infection or fungal problems a few weeks later. Yes, people with a fungus or "yeast infection" is also called "athlete's foot" or "athlete's itch" to name just a few types, but there are many other types of problems, related to fungi, that can come if your "good bacteria" and "bad bacteria" out of balance. In any case, plan to get a little per-biotika in the next week or two, when you are out of the antibiotic cycle. Take cabbage for dinner several times a week, or maybe give a little yogurt for breakfast. BTW, Pro-biotics mode, as found, to prevent "bird flu" and successfully treated, which should never burst and become a problem.

Last Thoughts:

The best solution is, of course, Preventive Medicine - take care of yourself first and foremost, do not get sick. No medicine will replace the right diet, rest, exercise, and preventive measures. Take your vitamins, lots of exercises, etc. antioxidants, etc. are a good way to boost the immune system, too slightly, but that's another debate.

If you liked this article and want to participate in other discussions about natural and alternative medicine, among a variety of other things, then you are invited to visit the mountain forum, where we dig around all aspects of the "mountain man "way of life.

Warning: as with any ongoing treatment, proceed with a little common sense. If (e) are properly educated before taking medications or supplements, or consult an Accredited Specialist, you can trust. Before starting treatment, make sure that it has been diagnosed correctly. Some people have allergies or intolerances to certain plants and chemicals, and these plants or chemicals are not suitable medicines for people. This article aims to educate your readers about the possibility of alternatives to frequent allopathic solutions. The author is not a health professional and should not be confused. Take the information here, explore for yourself, and use your best judgment on how to use it.

HERBAL ANTIFUNGAL REMEDIES

Antifungal and treatments are used to eradicate fungi and yeast that cause infections in many areas of the body.

These treatments are used to treat common conditions like athlete's foot, ringworm, dandruff, and vaginitis, as well as the difficult conditions that have spread throughout the body. Antifungal drugs are often used in people with a poorly functioning immune system, as is seen particularly in people with AIDS and those who are taking medications that suppress immune function.

Different Types of Fungal Infections

Here are some common types of fungal infections that affect and irritate many people.

- The athlete's foot is a type of fungal infection that usually appears between the toes but can also affect the toenails and the bottom or sides of the feet.

- Worm. This is a fungal infection of hair, skin, or nails. When it is on the skin, tinea usually begins as a small red area the size of a pea. As it grows, it stretches in a circle or circle. This infection is commonly called ringworm because it can look like small worms under the skin.

- Jock itch is a fungal infection of the groin and upper thighs and occurs in both men and women.

- Honest. This yeast infection is similar to a fungus. Usually, it affects the skin around the nails or soft and moist areas around the holes of the body. Diaper rash in children can be a candidias is type of infection. Older girls and women may develop another form of candidal infection in and around the vagina, and these are called yeast infections.

Herbal Antifungal Treatment

- Garlic. This herb is considered a strong antimicrobial substance. It was used by Albert Schweitzer to treat amoebic dysentery and also by Louis Pasteur as an antibacterial agent. Garlic is one of the richest sources of the element germanium, which is a strong inducer of interferon and effective against some tumors by modulating the immune response.

- Tea tree oil is an extract of the original tree, which is common in Australia. This is a cure for many fungal infections of the mucous membranes. Oil is used internally for thrush and esophagus, and externally for fungal infections of the skin and nail bed. Tea tree oil and grapefruit seed extract can be used for the external treatment of candida-related skin disease by 2-3 drops of each a lotion or balm and spreading it over the affected area.

- Oregano. The extract of this herb is considered stronger and less harmful than Nystatin to eradicate fungi. To eradicate staphylococcal infections, it is also considered more effective and less toxic.

- Echinacea is an immunostimulant and antiseptic plant. Scientific research shows herbal antibiotic activity similar to cortisone and helps to promote wound healing, production of systemic interferon, and stimulation of T lymphocytes.

- Pau d'arco. This herb is derived from an extract of the bark of a South American tree and is famous for its powerful antifungal properties.

- The Golden Seal. This herb is considered effective in treating most digestive problems ranging from peptic ulcers to colitis due to its tonic effects on the mucous membranes. It is a powerful antimicrobial substance that improves all mucous membranes, especially mucous membranes.

HERBAL HEMORRHOID REMEDIES

Hemorrhoids are a common problem, and millions of people around the world suffer from this disease. This is an old problem, and there is no reason to be ashamed of this problem. There are many remedies for hemorrhoids available, such as surgery, allopathic remedies, homeopathy, and herbal remedies. All these methods have cured the problem for thousands of people.

However, in recent years, herbal hemorrhoids drugs have gained great popularity. People choose herbal remedies instead of surgery or antibiotics. The main reason for this change is that these drugs provide relief from pain, itching, and inflammation caused by hemorrhoids. Popular herbs such as witch hazel, Butcher broom, Aloe vera, etc. have amazing results for sufferers without causing other health problems.

In addition, herbs used as remedies for hemorrhoids also help in the treatment of other diseases that a person may suffer from. Natural herbal ingredients are safe and often adapt well to the human body. These herbs are inexpensive and can be easily purchased at an herb store. The only drawback of herbs is that they do not need to bring immediate results.

Some herbs are used topically, and some can be used orally as hemorrhoid drugs. There are some herbs that can be applied locally and also consumed orally. For example, aloe vera can be applied to swollen veins, and it can also be consumed orally. The combination of treatment with herbal hemorrhoids usually gives excellent and long-lasting results.

Another advantage of herbal hemorrhoids is that this treatment may not be in the form of pills and ointments. Herbs can also be part of your diet by using them in cooking. There are many herbs such as mint, coriander, ginger, and cumin seeds that are used in cooking food. Some of these herbs will ease constipation and improve bowel movements.

BV HERBAL REMEDY

BV (or bacterial vaginosis) should be treated as soon as possible after a positive diagnosis. Either with the use of antibiotics or a herbal remedy BV, the elimination of BV will avoid other complications that can affect fertility and pregnancy. Herbal remedies for BV are now accepted as the most effective and less intrusive form of treatment.

The World Organization for women's health States: worldwide, a herbal remedy is now the most common remedy for BV. Also, in the United States, in 2008, just under 35% of women with bacterial vaginosis underwent an herbal remedy for their bacterial information.

Facts about BV and herbal remedy

BV is not a disease or something new that is introduced into the body. It is caused when anaerobes, a form of bacteria already present in the vagina, increase too much, and lactobacilli, another type of bacteria, decrease.

This balance causes a yellow/white film that adheres to the walls of the vagina and is periodically discharged, with a nauseating smell, especially after sexual intercourse. In addition to discharge and smell, patients experience intense vaginal itching.

Physical problems can check if the condition is left too long. Often the biggest problems are psychological. Women often feel embarrassed and form an adventure for sexual intercourse.

BV herbal remedies have a rate of clarification that approaches 100%, compared to 63%, with the use of antibiotics. They also tend to erase the condition forever, while there is a high rate of relapse with antibiotic remedies.

Another great advantage of an herbal remedy for BV is no side effects. Most of us are aware nowadays how much the immune system can be affected by the use of antibiotics. Herbal remedies, on the contrary, effectively help build the immune system while eradicating vaginitis at the same time.

Ingredients for an herbal remedy for BV should not cost more than four or five dollars. You need a good guide that explains the ingredients and preparation involved, as well as the amount and frequency of use.

Other good practices include drinking more water, not watering, keeping dry and clean, avoiding scented personal hygiene products, and avoiding slightly looser cotton jeans and underwear.

BV (bacterial vaginosis) needs treatment once it has been diagnosed by the patient or by a doctor or clinical counselor. BV natural remedies are the safest and safest ways to get rid of BV.

According to the Institute for women's health and wellness in Washington DC, just under 8% more women choose BV natural remedies year after year. The medical profession supports and encourages the use of BV herbal remedies, and soon the use of antibiotics as a treatment will be obsolete.

Bacterial vaginosis must participate, one way or another, because otherwise, it is capable of causing complications beyond this intense itching and horrible smell. Untreated infections of the fallopian tubes and / or uterus may occur.

Pelvic inflammatory disease is not uncommon in untreated BV patients. PID can lead to ectopic pregnancy and the inability to conceive. Abortions can occur if bacterial vaginosis is carried in pregnancy.

Of course, it is obvious that BV can also put a lot of women out of sex. It is usually at its worst after sexual intercourse, so victims often give up sex to avoid terrible itching and disgusting fish smells.

Why switch from antibiotics to alternative remedies for bacterial vaginosis?

Antibiotics can take place there and, until recently, were the de facto treatment of BV. However, metronidazole and clindamycin affect good bacteria that are vital for a healthy immune system. Treatment can be prolonged, and a woman's health often deteriorates with time.

BV natural remedies, on the other hand, do not have side effects and do not affect the natural balance of the body. The rate of clarification, especially if it is accompanied by a specific diet, is also much higher with BV natural remedies. The duration of treatment is also significantly shorter. In addition, the entire immune system is improved. Many women choose to continue a natural course because they get sick less frequently and feel better in general.

Most BV remedies cost only a few dollars for a month of supply. You simply know the ingredients, how, and in what quantities to mix and then, the way and frequency of intake.The basic advice boils down to get a proven guide BV natural remedies, so you know how to make the remedy, what foods to avoid, and what diet to follow. In addition to this, you should consider regular exercise and ways to reduce stress levels.

Kate Liberty

Herbal Antivirals

A Complete Guide to Discover the Secrets of Natural Remedies to Prevent and Cure Viral Infections with Medicinal Herbs

Copyright © 2020 publishing.

All rights reserved.

Author: Kate Liberty

No part of this publication may be reproduced, distributed or transmitted in any form or by any means, including photocopying recording or other electronic or mechanical methods or by any information storage and retrieval system without the prior written permission of the publisher, except in the case of brief quotation embodies in critical reviews and certain other non-commercial uses permitted by copyright law.

ANTIVIRAL HERBS

Antiviral herbs are part of the holistic approach to maintaining health. Unlike over-the-counter drugs such as antibiotics, which aim to eliminate infectious pathogens such as fungi and bacteria, antiviral herbs supplement the body's ability to heal itself even from supposedly incurable diseases.

Drugs are not only not natural, but also tend to work against the body. Chemical drugs work regardless of the body's natural functions and balances, which explains their long list of side effects. Another risk from the use of drugs is that viruses can become immune to their effects. In this condition, the next step is usually to take higher doses or use more powerful drugs that can pose a serious risk of damaging some organs and compromising the overall balance of the functions of the organ system.

While herbs are generally known for their culinary roles, there are some herbs that are established as natural remedies for viral infections. Their natural medicinal properties present excellent alternatives to common antiviral drugs. Unlike chemical drugs, these herbs safely provide a reliable defense against a whole spectrum of viruses.

Garlic is perhaps a centuries-old healing tool. It is also a powerful anti-pathogenic herb that can fight infectious viruses, bacteria, fungi, and other known pests. In some cases, fresh garlic juice is even more powerful than pharmaceutical antiviral drugs in that its healing properties can quickly penetrate into any part of the body, accelerate healing, and inhibit infection.

St. John's wort is presented as a healing herb. However, it is best known for its antiviral effects. Along with other powerful herbs such as garlic and Echinacea, it can form a powerful antiviral mixture.

Echinacea is an antiviral herb that fights infection by providing immunostimulating effects. In this sense, it helps double or even quadruple the number of immune cells and chemicals to reverse the functions of the immune system slow and optimize the body's defense against viral infections.

Goldenseal is another antiviral and antibacterial herb that offers a milder antiviral action, making it excellent for curing viral infections of sensitive parts of the body.

Other powerful antiviral herbs include oregano, Siberian Ginseng, astralago, peppermint, juniper, elderberry, burdock, and licorice. Astralagus is an effective antiviral remedy for viral disorders such as influenza and colds. Elderberry provides antiviral, antibacterial, and anti-inflammatory relief from colds, flu, and upper respiratory tract infections.

Antiviral herbs help overwhelm viruses by interfering with their replication cycle and inhibiting their activities. Usually, viruses attach to host cells where they interfere with natural cellular functions that cause infection or disease. Reference herbs have innate antiviral properties that are primarily designed to relieve and stimulate the functions of the immune system. In a sense, these herbs offer a naturally adaptable solution in which the body develops a strong defense against viral activities.

By stimulating the body's production of antiviral agents such as infection that fights white blood cells, antiviral herbs can significantly reduce the symptoms of infections and viral diseases. However, this does not necessarily mean that medicinal herbs alone can solve infections and viral diseases. A nutrient-rich and well-balanced diet is still needed to promote healing and better health.

There are many fantastic antiviral herbs. This is good news for those who want to take better care of their health and combat illness without the use of pharmaceuticals. Here we will talk about the best natural antiviral and their attributes.

Some of the best antiviral herbs include oregano, Echinacea, garlic, astragalus, schizandra, elderberry, mullein, licorice, and green tea.

* Oregano has been used for hundreds of years to fight viral, bacterial, and fungal infections. This is a well-known herb for seasoning food, particularly Italian dishes. However, this is a powerful foe against germs.

* Echinacea is well known for its ability to boost the immune system. It is said to stimulate white blood cell production, thus helping the body to fight viruses more effectively. This herb is best taken early on when an infection is first suspected, for the best results.

* Garlic is a very powerful antiviral herb that is very effective when used to fight the common cold and flu viruses as well as strep and staph infections. Garlic is wonderfully aromatic and is best consumed fresh, but it is also available in capsule and tablet form for those who want its health benefits without the garlic breath.

* Astragalus is another excellent immune strengthener and a very effective antiviral herb for combating the common cold and flu.

* Schizandra is one of the lesser-known herbal antivirals, which has been found to be very successful when treating viral hepatitis.

* Elderberry has been used as a herbal remedy against various viral infections for thousands of years. It is beneficial in fighting colds, flu, and upper respiratory infections. Typically, elderberry is most effective in lozenge and syrup form.

* Mullein provides antiviral, anti-inflammatory, calming, and expectorant properties, among other benefits. It is an excellent herbal choice for those suffering from congestion.

* Licorice is another excellent antiviral herb that is very effective against viruses and bacteria as well as fungal infections. Individuals with hypertension should avoid taking licorice.

* Green tea has been found effective in preventing the spread of the flu virus as well as promoting overall good

health due to its high levels of antioxidants and catechins ECG and EGCG.

Antiviral Essential Oils

Some wonderful antiviral essential oils include eucalyptus oil, tea tree oil, juniper oil, and lemon balm oil. These are helpful to use along with the above herbs when fighting a viral illness.

* Eucalyptus oil contains known antiviral compounds to help speed healing. Add a few drops of oil to a warm bath and breathe in the steam to help ease congestion. It can also be used in massage oil or applied to pulse points.

* Tea tree oil is another effective antiviral essential oil and can be applied full strength to external areas or gargled in water for sore throat.

* Juniper oil is a potent antiviral that has been found effective against herpes and flu viruses. It can be used in a diffuser, as a massage oil, or in a soothing bath.

* Lemon balm oil has many uses, including treatment of cold sores and genital sores caused by the herpes simplex virus and is effective for keeping the virus from spreading. Lemon balm oil can be used topically, in a diffuser, or taken internally.

THE USE OF ANTIVIRAL DRUGS-ALL YOU NEED TO KNOW

There are several reasons why people switch to herbal medicines, especially antiviral drugs, but of course, you need to be sure that the choice is right for you. One study shows that almost a third of Americans use herbal remedies and intend to continue doing so, but everyone should take into account the following conditions:

Other medicines you are taking-you should consult your doctor to check that there are no negative interactions.

Side effects-herbal preparations have a much lower probability of side effects than conventional antibiotics, but you should always be aware of what can happen.

Regulation-herbal preparations are not treated as follows:

There are a lot of resources and information that will help you make decisions, but some groups have not been tested properly: pregnant or lactating women, children, or the elderly. It is always better to consult your doctor first.

The Virus is described as:

"A large group of infectious agents which are sub-microscopic, which are considered micro-organisms, which need to be molecules of very simple or extremely complex, which typically contain a layer of proteins surrounding a core of RNA or DNA genetic material but no semi-permeable membrane, that is able to grow and multiply only in the body."

The Virus is not considered "alive" because it cannot replicate outside the host. Viruses penetrate and infect cells before using them to replicate and mutate, which can eventually kill cells. An example is the influenza virus that attacks the respiratory system.

It is difficult to produce safe and effective prescription antiviral drugs without damaging the cell used by the virus to replicate. The first experimental antiviral drugs were developed in 60 Years, thanks to methods of discovery by trial and error, originally intended for the herpes virus. Only 80 years, when they are obviously the complete genetic sequence of viruses, scientists can work to correct the chemicals needed to suppress their reproductive cycle.

"Antiviral drugs work biochemically, which allows propagation of the virus impossible," says Randy Wexler,

MD, assistant professor of Family Medicine at The Ohio State University College of Medicine in Columbus.

HOW HERBAL ANTIVIRAL DRUGS WORK

One of these ways is to break the replication cycle. Another way to work "antiviral" in order to stimulate the immune system. Antiviral drugs can bind to certain enzymes and prevent adsorption on the host cell.

Michael Moore, a herbalist, describes antiviral drugs in his medical glossary:

"A substance that experimentally suppresses the spread and vitality of infectious viruses. In our field of medicinal plants, some plants slow or inhibit the adsorption or random initial fixation of viruses to prolong the life of infected target cells or to accelerate various aspects of immunity, including responses to complement, antibodies, and phagocytosis. Herbal antivirals work best on respiratory viruses such as influenza, adenoviruses, rhinoviruses, and enteric echoviruses. Presented as useful in the alphabet group of slow viruses (HIV, EBV, CMV, etc.), they really help to reduce concomitant secondary respiratory infections, which often accompany immunosuppression." Of course, there are advantages and disadvantages to traditional antiviral and herbal drugs.

TRADITIONAL ANTIVIRAL DRUGS

Advantages:

- They help you overcome a viral infection faster.
- It is easy to take them often in the form of tablets or capsules.
- Traditional medicines are controlled by the governing body to ensure their safety.

Disadvantages:

- Side effects include nausea, vomiting, cough, runny/stuffy nose, diarrhea.
- They are not indispensable; One will recover from a viral infection without them.

HERBAL ANTIVIRALS DRUGS

Advantages:

- Herbal antiviral drugs provide much fewer side effects.
- It costs much less, and it's easier to get to them.

Disadvantages:

- There is no herbal antiviral regulation, which means that it can be difficult to find all the necessary information.
- They may interact with other medications you are taking.

There are several ways your body can fight infections and naturally strengthen your immune system; it's designed to do it. Sometimes it just needs a little help when it comes to viruses. In addition to herbal remedies, there are factors that you can include in your daily lifestyle as a preventive method:

- Do not smoke.
- Eat healthy diets, fruits, vegetables, whole grains, and low saturated fat.
- Practice.
- Maintain a healthy weight.

- Check your blood pressure.
- If you drink alcohol, do it in moderation.
- Sleep well.
- Take measures to prevent infection, often wash your hands, carefully cook meat, etc.
- Get regular medical screening tests tailored to your age and risk group.

ANTIVIRAL HERBS FOR QUICK AND SAFE RELIEF

Antiviral herbs are part of a holistic approach to maintaining health. Unlike over-the-counter drugs, such as antibiotics, whose purpose is to eliminate infectious pathogens, such as fungi and bacteria, antiviral herbs supplement the body's ability to cure even seemingly incurable diseases.

Drugs are not only not natural, but also tend to work against the body. Chemical drugs work independently of the natural functions and balance of the body, which explains their long list of side effects. Another risk of taking medications is that viruses can become immune to their effects. In this condition, the next stage is usually the use of higher doses or the use of stronger drugs that can pose a serious risk of harm to some organs and stop the general balance of the functions of the authority.

While herbs are generally known for their culinary roles, some herbs are established as natural remedies for viral infections. Their natural healing properties are an excellent alternative to conventional antiviral drugs. Unlike chemical drugs, these herbs safely provide a reliable defense against the entire spectrum of viruses.

Garlic is perhaps a centuries-old healing tool. It is also a strong anti-pathogenic plant that can fight infectious viruses, bacteria, fungi, and other known pests. In some cases, fresh garlic juice is even more powerful than pharmaceutical antiviral drugs in that its healing properties can quickly penetrate into any part of the body, accelerate healing, and suppress infection.

St. John's wort is offered as a medicinal herb. However, it is best known for its antiviral effects. Along with other strong herbs such as garlic and Echinacea, it can create a powerful antiviral mixture.

Echinacea is an antiviral herb that fights infection by providing immunostimulating effects. In this sense, it helps to double or even quadruple the number of immune cells and chemicals to reverse the function, slow down the immune system and optimize the body's defenses against viral infections.

Goldenseal is another antiviral and antibacterial herb that offers a milder antiviral action, making it excellent for treating viral infections of sensitive parts of the body.

Other powerful antiviral herbs include oregano, Siberian ginseng, astragalus, peppermint, juniper, elderberry, burdock, and licorice. Astralagus is an effective antiviral drug for viral ailments such as influenza and colds. Elderberry berries provide antiviral, antibacterial, and anti-inflammatory relief from colds, flu, and upper respiratory tract infections.

Antiviral herbs help overwhelm viruses by interfering with their replication cycle and inhibiting their activities. Viruses usually attach to host cells where they interfere with natural cellular functions that cause infection or disease. Reference herbs have innate antiviral properties, which are primarily designed to relieve and stimulate the function of the immune system. In a sense, these herbs offer a naturally adaptable solution in which the body develops a strong defense against viral activities.

By stimulating the body's production of antiviral agents such as infection that fights white blood cells, antiviral herbs can significantly reduce the symptoms of infections and viral diseases. However, this does not necessarily mean that the treatment of the herbs themselves can solve infections and viral diseases. Nutritionally, a rich and balanced diet, is always needed to promote healing and better health.

NATURALLY STRENGTHEN THE IMMUNE SYSTEM WITH ANTIVIRAL HERBS

The human immune system is a complex process, which protects our health and provides protection against viruses, bacteria, microbes, parasites, and toxins. Antiviral herbs support the body's natural ability to stay in a healthy balance and naturally strengthen the immune system, which is the first line of defense against diseases and diseases.

Conventional antibiotics are not an effective defense against viruses and, if taken unnecessarily, can be counterproductive.

Numerous clinical research studies have confirmed traditional medicine that takes herbal medicines after a certain period of time to promote the health and vitality and benefits of herbs. Some of these herbs that develop the immune system are:

Abstract Olive Leaf is known to support healthy phagocytosis, the purpose of the immune system in which phagocytes into the bloodstream probably pass harmful microorganisms.

Research has shown that African potato extract has positive effects on the number of T-lymphocytes involved in improving immunity.

Buchu promotes the body's ability to get rid of harmful toxins through the urinary system.

Peppermint helps to strengthen liver function by promoting the natural flow of bile into the body. Mint oils are useful for promoting a healthy immune system.

The Golden Rod strengthens the body's natural protective ability to fight infections and regulate the production of mucus.

Research has shown that the European mistletoe promotes a natural immune response and helps maintain a balanced level of fluid in the body and strengthens the walls of the capillaries.

Hawthorn is highly respected in herbal medicine as a tonic to promote healthy circulation. Research studies have shown the ability of Hawthorn to help with heart function.

Wu Wei Zi (Schizandra Sinesis) - studies show that this Chinese herb can help support the healthy function of the heart, liver, and kidneys.

Seeded milk is a Chinese herb that is known to have positive effects on the health and functioning of the immune system.

More frequent attacks of colds, flu, and other minor infections are more likely if you have problems with immunity. Although antibiotics can be miracle drugs, they should not be considered a "quick fix." And as mentioned above, they are not effective against viruses.

Antiviral herbs act to strengthen your immune system so that your body can naturally and easily protect itself from anything you might encounter.

THE BEST SOURCES FOR HERBAL ANTIVIRAL DRUGS

Herbal antiviral drugs can be found everywhere. They are not necessarily purchased in the form of a supplement. In fact, including antiviral foods in your daily diet is a great way to help prevent viruses, which affect you.

They are considered the best natural antiviral drugs in foods, herbs, and spices such as:

Cat's claw

Cranberry

Senior

Ginger

Melissa

Licorice Root

Of Olive Leaves

Oregano

These herbs are designed as the best antiviral herbs:

Turmeric

Cinnamon

Garlic

Oregano

Rosemary

Ginger

Mint

Basil

COMMON VIRAL INFECTIONS AND THEIR CAUSES

Most viral infections disappear over time; however, this does not mean that the virus is no longer in your body. Viruses affect any part of the body or body system, which leads to infections such as:

Colds are one of the most common infections. It is accompanied by symptoms such as sore throat, fever, cough, and sometimes stuffy nose. Its duration varies from two days to two weeks on a more serious note. It is very portable and can be easily transmitted from person to person, especially in a poorly ventilated room. A person can suffer from colds several times a year.

Viral infections on the skin are also possible leading to warts or chickenpox. They have an itchy rash, migraine, and fever. It spreads through the behavior of the skin with an infected person. It is mild and lasts no more than two weeks, although, in adults, it can be of moderate severity. A person suffers from chickenpox only once in his life. It is similar to measles and smallpox, although they are treated with various medications.

Headache, sore throat, fever, and muscle aches are examples of the symptoms of influenza, often called influenza. Unlike other viral infections can cause serious and sometimes fatal complications, but they can be treated easily and economically.

Viruses can cause infections of the gastrointestinal system, causing inflammation of the intestine (gastroenteritis). This is mainly about the unhealthy manipulation of food and the inability to wash your hands after visiting the toilet or after changing baby diapers.

Human papilloma virus (HPV) is one of the most common sexually transmitted viruses. This is the cause of genital warts. Other common sexually transmitted viruses are herpes and HIV.

There is another infection called a cold that has flu-like symptoms. The only difference is the appearance of ulcers on the sides of the mouth, which are rather unattractive. Insects are also known to transmit viruses such as yellow fever and dengue.

COMMON NATURAL ANTIVIRAL HERBS

There are hundreds of herbs known to show a significant amount of antiviral activity when used. They can be readily available in your garden or local market, while others can be very difficult to find. It is recommended to consult an expert on herbal products, to achieve the right dosage and conditions of use. For example, some herbs should not be taken during pregnancy. Also, remember that most of the indicated herbs are used to treat more than one viral infection. Some are also strong enough to kill all other harmful pathogens. It is also possible to find an infection that has more than one natural remedy.

Olive leaf can be used in tea with mint or as a capsule. Most often, it is used in the treatment of influenza, colds, and herpes.

Melissa: This is another herb rich in antiviral properties. It is used in the treatment of gastric diseases and skin infections when applied topically. For oral administration, you can make an infusion (add warm water). It is believed that it is not suitable for use during pregnancy.

Adding ginger to tea and food is not only tastier, but it is also known to prevent and reduce the time it takes to disappear colds. It also relieves pain in the neck and chest. When mixed with honey, this is a strong herb in the treatment of influenza and the reduction of sore throat. It can also be crushed or cut into small pieces and added to warm water.

Chlorella: Chlorella is a small unicellular green alga, which is not only an impressive source of nutrition but is also known to improve the immune system. A strong immune system helps fight viruses, thereby preventing infection or preventing the spread of infection.

Chamomiles: Chamomiles are used to make herbal infusions for medical purposes. This daisy-like plant is the treatment of gastrointestinal disorders and relieves inflammation and ulcers. Preference is given to the removal of crushed juice, which is added to warm water.

Cayenne Pepper: These are undoubtedly one of the most powerful herbs in the world. It has many medicinal values, is the treatment and relief of colds, sore throat, stomach pain, and prevents the emergence of other pathogens, such as fungi. It is added to food as a spice.

Cranberry: It is not only used for its culinary activities, but in fact, it is a powerful medicinal plant. It is used to treat disorders that occur in the gastrointestinal system and circulatory complications. Fruit juice is drunk in a full or half-full cup. It is sweet, so you do not need to add sweetener, as in the case of other herbs.

The weed, commonly known as Black-bunched Acea, is used to treat kidney infections and sore throat. The grass is squeezed and drunk for a few days. However, the herb has serious side effects, such as dizziness, headaches, cramps, nausea, vomiting, sweating, and low blood pressure.

Chili: This has been used in traditional medicine for centuries, especially in Asian countries such as India. It is used to treat herpes and other respiratory infections. It is used in food or applied locally by adding water or milk and is one of the most commonly used spices in the world.

Garlic: A Garlic is an indisputable traditional medicine. It is used as a remedy for various diseases, including warts, flu, and colds. There are other natural ways to treat genital warts, for example, when wet oats or putting onion slices on warts. However, the onion is not sufficiently scientifically proven. I advise you to consult your doctor because these drugs treat only warts, not HPV, which caused warts. They say that chewing raw garlic helps patients with high blood pressure. Most people use garlic as a dish, although it leaves a smell that does not disappear easily.

Astalagal Root: It is used as a preventive measure against influenza. It works best by increasing the body's immune system, which allows the body to fight viruses. It is recommended to take it in anticipation of the onset of the disease flu season, not when you already have it. Use it in herbal tea or cooked in food.

Cat Pike: Cat Pike, taken in a capsule or tea, is a strong antiviral, antibacterial and antifungal herb. It is also a powerful stimulant of the immune system.

We cannot talk about herbs without mentioning aloe vera. It is a herb that heals almost everything. It's from the same family as agave. It is very bitter and may require additional sweetener; preference is given to honey. It can be administered orally or locally and is considered very effective.

Roots, leaves, seeds, and berries of the elderberry tree are used to treat colds and flu. Due to the high level of cyanide present in the plant, it is necessary to completely boil it before use as a medicinal product.

Oregano Oil: Oregano oil is used as a medicine and as a flavor in food. These are antiviral drugs, as it speeds up the healing process and prevents skin irritation when used locally.

Licorice Root: This is used as a tea and drunk on their own or can be mixed with other herbal tea in the treatment of gastric ulcers. It is both an antibacterial and antiviral.

COMMON BACTERIAL INFECTION

Most of the bacteria present in the human body are not harmful; on the contrary, they are very beneficial. It is believed that only 1% of bacteria in our body are harmful. The rest is useful to help digestion and other important functions of the body. Some of the bacteria are also known to prevent cancer risk and help in the respiratory and urinary tract.

Unlike viruses, living micro-organisms are bacteria that can live and reproduce without being attached to a living cell. They are even bigger than viruses.

Common Bacterial Infections

It is known that not all bacteria are harmless and beneficial; some are very harmful and can have a significant impact on a person's health. Some of these infections include tuberculosis, which affects millions of people, especially in sub-Saharan Africa. It is very contagious and airborne. It affects the respiratory system, including the lungs, and can kill if it is not detected and treated in time.

Other common bacterial infections include typhoid, tetanus, syphilis, pneumonia, Hansen's disease, dental cavities, gingivitis, epiglottitis, tonsillitis, Legionnaires ' disease, pertussis, anthrax, and meningitis.

There are bacteria transmitted by dangerous sex. These include syphilis, chlamydia, and gonorrhea. These infections are treatable. Early diagnosis and treatment are recommended to prevent other complications, such as pelvic inflammatory diseases.

Prostatitis is a bacterial infection that affects the prostate in men. In women, some bacteria responsible for urinary tract infections.

Antibiotics At Home

Antibiotics can also be called antibacterial drugs. Pharmaceutical antibiotics come from certain types of fungi. They are used to treat bacterial infections. People who take antibiotics know that drug resistance develops, that is, the drugs cannot work when taken.

Most pharmaceutical antibiotics prescribed by doctors may show signs of side effects such as nausea, dizziness, and vomiting, in some cause allergic reactions, such as skin rashes or itching; some can also kill the good bacteria that help in certain body functions. We cannot exclude side effects when using natural substances; however, there are fewer possible side effects, and most are manageable.

There are millions of people who are allergic to certain herbs: some people are allergic to nuts, others to honey, and others may be allergic to berries. One of the advantages of using natural remedies is that it is common to find more than one natural treatment for an infection. In this case, you can choose the one to which you are not allergic. Let's look at the common natural antibiotics that are available to treat infections.

Garlic and onions have been used for their antibacterial and antiviral capabilities since time immemorial. It is believed that they help reduce inflammation and reduce the risk of developing hypertension and stroke.

It has been proved that any food rich in vitamin C, contains antibacterial and antiviral properties. They strengthen the body's immunity, force the body to defend itself, and also help the speed of healing. The main sources of vitamin C are fruits such as strawberries, lemons and limes, pineapples, watermelons and oranges, and most vegetables, such as broccoli, tomatoes, spinach, and cabbage. Kiwi is not only rich in vitamin C, but it is also supposed to contain all other essential nutrients. This is the best fruit for all its nutrients, and also one of the most expensive fruit.

Eucalyptus produces a powerful antiseptic that kills most pathogens, including bacteria. It is added to tea and gives a wonderful taste.

Some bacteria are transmitted through the food we eat. Use horseradish in the food you eat. Bacteria are killed even before they enter the body. It is used as a vegetable.

Coconut oil contains an important substance known as lauric acid. Its main function is to dissolve pathogens. Oil can be used in the preparation of dishes, or oil can be drunk alone.

Scientists have suggested using fermented foods such as fermented vegetables to help deliver good bacteria to the body. These foods are known as probiotics and are recommended to be used with antibiotics.

It is known that the marshmallow root has properties that relieve pain. It is also effective for killing bacteria in the urinary tract. The preparation is best taken orally in the form of infusion (with warm water). Another herb that can be used to treat urinary tract infections is Yarrow. It is also used as a tea. It is not recommended to use it during pregnancy, as it can cause uterine contractions.

Turmeric is a very strong medicinal plant, which is usually crushed to form a yellow/orange powder. It is used to treat various bacterial, fungal, and viral infections.

NATURAL REMEDIES FOR THE TREATMENT OF ALLERGIES

Millions of people around the world suffer from allergies. Allergies are negative reactions of a person's body to a particular substance. People are allergic to many things, some of the most common allergies include, protein allergies caused by pollen, as well as some people are allergic to certain tissues, nuts, honey, Cats, Dogs, dust, cold and many others.

Allergies are often characterized by effects, itching, and congestion. There are many drugs that relieve alternatives and itching, but almost none that reduces congestion. Most of these drugs are also expensive and have side effects such as drowsiness and irritation of the nose. Most natural remedies have fewer side effects, if any; however, they only work by preventing energy from occurring.

The simplest form of prevention is to rinse with water as soon as possible after contact with electricity. Salt can be added to the water to effectively rinse the pollen grains.

Eating free foods containing omega-3 reduces the likelihood that a person will suffer from allergic reactions. Common foods with omega-3 are; fish, eggs, and linseed oil. The use of horseradish, chili, and heated Mustard could also help to temporarily decongest.

There are natural antihistamines that work, one is nettle and the other is PetaSite. These natural remedies have an advantage over drugs that have no side effects.

If you are allergic to certain foods, you can completely eliminate them. If this is not possible, there is an unorthodox method that can be used even if it is risky, and there are no known chances of success. It is about consuming food to which you are allergic more often; it is believed by some people that this makes the body accustomed to food. This method is not recommended because it can cause severe allergic reactions.

TO IMPROVE IMMUNITY, USE PROVEN HERBAL REMEDIES

If a person suffers from a problem of immunity, then more frequent attacks of influenza, colds and minor infections are more likely. Antibiotics are very effective and high drugs, but their unscrupulous use is not recommended. Weak immunity is learned or primary. This condition is mainly due to a genetic predisposition. Weak immunity is an acquired condition that is affected by lifestyle, diet, and drug abuse in diseases, such as colds and more.

Our first line of defense against invaders like bacteria, pathogens, parasites, viruses, and more, is our immune system. To improve the immune system, natural and herbal remedies should be used. The construction of this complex system must be part of our daily routine. It is a fact that herbal antibiotics, a natural diet, and an active lifestyle are responsible for improving the health of our immune system and also help to prevent the disease, such as common and simple joint the daring and also the risk of diseases, such as cancer. Some of the common treatments to improve immunity are

1. Garlic is very effective and the oldest herb for improving the immune system. This is the oldest cultivated plant in the world. It has a history of strengthening the immune

system and as an effective herbal antibiotic from the days when the pyramids were built. They say that one of the most important elements of the immune system is the manufacturer of natural white blood cells.

2. Some vegetables that are red, orange, dark green, and carrots contain carotenoids, which are converted to vitamin-a by the liver. The latter is very effective and useful for thymus. Thymus plays an important role in the production of immunity. It is also useful in the Prevention of atrophy due to old age.

3. Zinc is also very effective in improving immunity. Some important and excellent sources of zinc are peanuts, peanut butter, dark chicken, lamb, and beef.

4. One of the important herbs for immunity is Ashwagandha. It is responsible for the stimulating effect on the immune system.

5. To maintain a healthy immune system, vitamins A, C, and E. We can get enough vitamin E from a handful of almonds a day. Natural sources of vitamin C are oranges and other citrus fruits. They are very effective in improving our immunity.

HOW TO USE MEDICINAL HERBS

Treatment with herbal remedies is controversial in the medical world. You can find doctors and pharmacologists who are against this completely citing the lack of scientific studies and unknown side effects. On the other hand, you can find holistic and homeopathic professionals who promote the wonders that nature has provided for the healing of all the diseases of the world. Natural food stores and vitamin suppliers are full of our shopping centers, and our shopping center is ready to "sell" the latest natural miracle herbs on the market today.

The truth lies somewhere between these rationalizations. A healthy body, mind, and spirits are much more complicated than taking "natural" pills or "the pill" prescribed to correct any disease we have. As part of the treatment can be the use of medicinal herbs if these herbs are used as teas, tonics, packages, packages, oils, or creams. An important factor, as with anything in life, is balance. We live in a world that rotates around the corner and wants to return to natural ways, whether it's "green" with our cars and homes or a return to natural and herbal remedies for our body.

Part of the balance in using medicinal herbs is the effort of your healthcare team. Explain to your health professionals, that your desire to work with a holistic approach to traditional medicine is the beginning, including changing the diet, which implements many common herbs that can be used in a culinary environment to promote a healthier body, as well as food for the mind and thoughts.

To begin with, there are some medicinal herbs that present a very low health risk when using, which can start anyone on the way to finding a balance in the use of herbs with other aspects of healthy living.

* Aloe vera juice is an antiseptic of nature and is used as a basis in many products sold on the market today. When used externally, no one can doubt its healing properties.

* Thyme-tasting herbaceous clover used in many French dishes. When brewing tea from thyme, it is believed that it helps to relieve swelling, headaches, inflammation, asthma, whooping cough, and stomach cramps.

* Chives-a more delicate sweet onion flavor is used in a variety of culinary dishes. As with all herbs, from the onion family, its hot vapors can eliminate congestion, and they are also said to help reduce blood pressure.

* Sage - this lemongrass with aromas is widely used in many dishes. In Germany, it is used as an antibiotic. This can help dry-milk nursing mothers faster when they are ready to breastfeed.

* Spicy-there are two varieties of spicy, and both are used in culinary recipes. Saturn is considered a mild disinfectant, and tea can be used for occasional diarrhea, minor stomach problems, and neck pain.

* Tarragon-a favorite herb in French cuisine, this herb can also be used to stimulate taste, and some believe that to help rheumatism. In herbs, there are also antioxidants.

* Garlic-most realize the taste of garlic and are well poured into its culinary use. Recently, it has been proved that the healing effects of this plant are excellent. Herbalists will tell you that garlic kills germs and is a natural antibiotic against influenza, viral infections, and yeast. It is a traditional remedy for worms in animals and humans. This can help with respiratory problems, as well as with hypertension. Chinese studies show that garlic can prevent certain types of stomach cancer. Herbalists believe that it is also useful for colds, infections of the kidneys, and bladder.

* Mint-there are several varieties and flavors of mint all for culinary use. Peppermint is a source of menthol and is therefore used in various traditional medicines. It also acts as an antispasmodic for the digestive systems and relieves spasms of the menstrual cycle.

* Oregano-better known in Italian cuisine, it is also thoughtful when the leaves are used in tea to relieve indigestion, cough, and headache. Grass oil works miracles when gout is placed on the tooth, which is painful.

* Persil-delicate flavor works well to mix other flavors together. The drug, of course, is the vitamin therapy itself, containing more vitamin C in volume than Orange. It also contains vitamin A, several B vitamins, calcium, and iron.

* Basil has long been used in culinary dishes because it is rich and spicy to taste. It can be used raw or dried. Basil is a member of the mint family and has long been used for digestive problems, as well as having a slight sedative action (perhaps that is why after a big Italian dinner, a nap sounds good).

* Cumin-each part of the cumin is edible. It is a spicy, nutty flavor and can be added to anything. It also has a property that helps with complaints of indigestion.

* Cloves - with its strong wintergreen-like flavor, cloves are commonly used in different cooking dishes. From the medical point of view, it has mild anesthetic properties and is usually recommended by a dentist for those who have sensitive teeth.

* Dill has a flavor mainly used to make cucumbers. It is known that swelling is also distracted. Interestingly, in pregnant women, it can stimulate milk production and increase appetite.

* Marjoram - similar to oregano, is used in various recipes. It is believed that marjoram has antioxidant and antifungal properties.

* Ginger tasting almost like citrus is used in various dishes. It relieves digestive problems and can prevent damage.

* Rosemary-it is difficult to describe the taste of rosemary, but from there, it says that it is robust. It is thought to help with various ailments, improves mood, headaches, muscle spasms, expectorant and leaves rubbed into the skin, it is thought to help with rheumatism and eczema.

* Cayenne pepper-if you are looking for a hot flash, this is the herb for you. Although these herbs are warm for taste buds, they have several medicinal properties. Ripe pepper

has more vitamin C than anything else you can grow in a garden at 369 milligrams per ounce. It also has a high content of vitamin A, iron, potassium, and niacin. Strangely enough, this burning substance helps to cleanse the digestive system, repel colds, and fever.

* Fennel-fennel leaves are commonly used in salads and seasonings in the sweet variety of herbs. It also has a weak diuretic property, and also a slight stimulus. It is also planned to increase the flow of milk in nursing mothers. An interesting banal fact: in medieval times, fennel was one of the nine sacred herbs that were considered to cure the nine causes of medieval diseases.

* Anise - a form of licorice, which can be used whole or ground. Leaves can be chopped and added to salads or try to make tea. Anise can improve digestion and prevent bloating. It's also thought that anise oil was a sweet hope.

* Cinnamon-a favorite in baking sweets, this herb can also help fight a number of fungi and bacteria, such as staphylococcal infections. It is also used to relieve vomiting.

In any case, this is not a complete list of common herbs used in culinary dishes that also have medicinal value. This is just the beginning, which shows that many herbs used in cooking can be added to our healthy lifestyle plan. All these herbs are considered completely safe and cause little or no side effects when used in moderation. Thinking about moving to a healthier lifestyle, consult your doctor, and look for a reliable holistic or homeopathic professional work.

THE BENEFITS OF GROWING MEDICINAL HERBS

If you have a garden, growing medicinal herbs gives you a wide range of benefits, all for the price of planting some unpleasant seeds! Let's look at some of the main advantages of growing medicinal plants outdoors.

Health

Even if you are a bigger user of traditional medicine than alternative medicine, there is no reason not to accept even the most subtle health benefits of herbs. Herbs have been used for their medicinal properties for thousands of years, and especially for minor problems and for stimulating the immune system, they are difficult to beat.

Here are some of the best herbs to grow for medicinal purposes: Echinacea (helps to activate white blood cells, helps the body fight infections, can protect against viral infections, such as colds); milk thistle (proven in many scientific studies, which help regulate and strengthen liver function), ginseng (lowers cholesterol and has a protective effect on the liver), ginseng (reduces cholesterol and has a protective effect

In general, the easiest way to take medicinal herbs, infusions. About ¼ cup of loose fresh herbs per cup of boiling water, it will usually give you enough strength to drink, as soon as you let it brew for 10-15 minutes (you can always set a different time if it is too strong or too weak). If you find unpleasant herbs, try adding lemon flavor, herbal mixtures, and also a little honey.

Durable, attractive and easy to grow plants for your garden

Most medicinal herbs are very unpretentious and easy to grow. Some of them are actually too easy to grow, and if uncontrolled, can take control of the garden! They are also very resistant to pests because the purpose of their essential oils is to repel insects (and discourage animals from eating them).

Personal satisfaction

Medicinal herbs have obvious advantages. But in addition to these (healthy qualities and aesthetic characteristics), growing herbs organically in your garden, and then collecting and using is improving the health of you and your family is just a pretty hard feeling to beat. There is no reason why you could not buy herbal medicines from the shop and grow flowers in your garden, but doing it yourself (and killed two pigeons with a bean) is very satisfying. Try it!

People grow medicinal herbs throughout human history. The use of medicinal herbs is mentioned in many ancient texts, including, for example, the Bible and the Koran. Even if they are not a substitute for traditional medicine, medicinal herbs can treat common ailments; you can boost your immune system, looks great in your garden, and provide you with a satisfying pastime as well.

VIRAL INFECTIONS, THE IMMUNE SYSTEM AND ANTIVIRAL SUPPLEMENTS

Now that summer is behind us, and the weather is cooler, we are sure that an increase in the number of colds, chills, and other viral infections is occurring. For most of us, winter is a little depressing disadvantage, which in the worst-case keeps us in bed for a day or two, but for the elderly and sick, a simple viral infection like a cold can leave you open to the attack of several dangerous diseases.

Many people wonder why there are no medications for colds and flu. With all that, modern medicine can certainly, given the treatment of such simple diseases as colds, it should be easy. The problem is not that we do not understand how viruses like colds and flu work (we understand them perfectly), but how quickly they mutate, that is, how quickly one type of cold can turn into another.

Let's start with what a virus is. The viruses have been maliciously described by a biologist as "a small piece of genetic code wrapped in bad news."Viruses are not technically alive - they have no cells or all the machines needed to support life and are completely parasitic. Viruses work simply by entering a living cell (depending on the virus, maybe bacteria, plant cells, fungal cells, or animal cells, such as a human cell) and essentially taking control of the machinery as a cell. The cell is then forced to produce multiple copies of the virus until there are so many copies that the cell bursts and all small copies are free to attack nearby cells.

Viruses are extremely simple. A typical virus contains only a small length of DNA or RNA (genetic material) enclosed in a hard protein layer (the bad news). This protein layer is a very specific form, and this is what allows the virus to penetrate the cells. That is, the protein layer binds to the structures on the attacking cell surface, allowing the virus (or at least its genetic material) to enter the cell. Once inside, the genetic material of the virus takes control of the cell, and millions of new copies are produced.

For the most part, these copies are identical to the original virus, but from time to time (about one copy in a billion), a mutation occurs. Since the order of its genes determines the form of the protein layer of the virus, a slight change in the genetic order caused by a single mutation can lead to viruses that have a different form of the protein layer. Most of these mutations will have layers that are now useless (the wrong shape to bind to cells), but some will have a layer of different shapes, allowing them to bind to different structures on their host cells. This newly mutated virus will spread and create more copies, and we have a new strain of the virus. This is really an evolution in action.

Therefore, it is unlikely that we will find a definitive "cure" for colds and other common viruses. You may be surprised to find yourself sheltered from the cold you've never experienced. When your body encounters a virus that is already infected, you can recognize it and destroy, but because viruses like colds are constantly mutating, there are always new types of colds, which you have already met, and you're always at risk of infection

Therefore, it is a good idea to make sure that the immune system works as efficiently as possible. The immune system is an incredibly complex and powerful set of tools that our body uses to defend itself against infections and destroy invasive viruses or bacteria. It works on different levels, but it is easier to consider when it comes to small permanent armies of different specialized cells. These cells protect your body, identify intruders like viruses, and try to destroy them. When a new invasive virus is found, the immune system must first find the protein molecules in the right form, or antibodies that destroy viruses, and this can take several days. Meanwhile, the virus generates billions of copies of itself, spreads through the system, and starts making you sick.

Perhaps it is surprising that the viruses themselves often do not get sick, but the body's efforts to destroy them. Having found the type of antibodies, it turned out that the immune system of the package, millions, and millions of copies, and uses a lot of energy, which leads to fatigue is a frequent symptom of the flu.

Strengthening the immune system and making sure that it has all the vitamins and minerals it needs to function effectively, can significantly reduce the risk of disease. If the immune system can quickly identify and destroy new invaders before the infection spreads, we can deal with viral infections, sometimes without even realizing it. In other words, you have a cold, and it will allow you to overcome without being sick.

Antiviral supplements contain vitamins and herbs that stimulate and support the immune system. When the body produces antibodies and immune cells, it uses a lot of vitamin C and zinc, and taking a daily supplement containing these substances can help keep the immune system functioning properly. The antiviral supplement also usually contains powerful antioxidants such as elderberry extract. Antioxidants help reduce the damage caused by so-called "free radicals" chemicals that are often produced as a by-product of the disease that attacks healthy cells. And finally, most antiviral supplements also contain Echinacea extract, which has been shown in some studies (others were less conclusive) to stimulate the production of immune cells and antibodies.

Antiviral supplements alone do not replace a healthy diet and healthy lifestyle, but they can help promote optimal functioning of the immune system and ensure that your body is ready to deal with any new invader more effectively than it otherwise would have been.

SINUSITIS HERBS

Sinusitis herbs have made a strong comeback as a way to treat breast problems. Ever-increasing industrialization has its advantages, but there are also disadvantages. Although diseases like smallpox are no longer ulcers, the increase in technology helped create the new, to support, and all other drugs. The disease occurred rarely, and therefore rest and recovery were the solutions. Today, diseases can last for years. Some diseases occur after a sick person hits the trigger. Asthma is one of them, and sinusitis is the other. Natural remedies and herbs are now sought by many to help relieve symptoms or cure the problem.

The use of herbs for the treatment of sinusitis has obvious advantages. One of them is their absence of side effects. The second is that they are quite inexpensive, and you can often find them in your kitchen or garden. The third is that they work not only to reduce symptoms but also to emphasize the underlying cause.

There are several herbs that can help prevent inflammation and increase the effectiveness of the immune system. Unicariaguianensis, known as Cat's claw, is one of these herbs. This plant is a remedy for colds and sinusitis. Recent research shows that it contains phytochemicals that deter bacterial and viral infections. The bark of the plant is what the herbalist uses to treat.

Astralagusmembranaceus, commonly called the astralagus and used in ancient Chinese medicine, has now turned out to be really effective due to the high content of zinc, potassium, calcium, manganese, and magnesium. These building blocks increase the effectiveness of the immune system in the fight against infections. The herb is also associated with drugs for lupus, rheumatoid arthritis, kidney disease, and diseases of the genitourinary system.

Another herb that helps is a redhead. It contains allicin, which eliminates the accumulation of blocked mucus. Ginger tea, a well-known treatment, can significantly improve the condition of the breast.

Echinacea, another of the popular herbs of sinusitis, is another excellent remedy. It is useful for those who experience side effects prescribed by a doctor and outside antidecongestants. It relieves symptoms and also decongests the head. You can take it in the form of capsules or drink as tea with honey and lemon.

You can't feel complete relief about taking pot.

A healthy lifestyle improves any treatment. No matter how many herbs use sinusitis, the effects are suppressed by poor life choices.

Possible Sinusitis Herbs

According to UMM, there are ways to use this herb for adults and children. For adults, you can use 1-2 grams of dried root or herbs as a tea, 2-3 ml of extract, tincture, standardized, 6-9 ml of expressed Juice, Juice), 300 mg of standardized extract powder containing 4% phenol dye (1: 5): 1 - 3 mL (20-90 drops), or stabilized fresh extract: 0.75 mL(15-23 drops). Choose one and take it three times a day for a week or ten days.

For children, it is necessary to adjust the dosage for adults to the weight of the child. The dose for adults is designed for an adult weighing 150 pounds. If the child weighs 50 pounds, the appropriate dose would be 1/3 of the adult dose.

Before using this herb, you should always consult your doctor. Although it is generally safe, there are reports of allergic reactions or drug interactions, which can lead to undesirable complications.

Barberry

Another ancient herb, dating from almost 2500 years ago, barberry is traditionally used in Indian folk medicine for diarrhea. Today it is used to relieve inflammation and infection of different parts of the body, including the respiratory tract (which could include the cavity).

Barberry is available in capsules, liquid extracts, tinctures, and in the form of local ointment.

According to UMM, it is not recommended to use this herb on children, since there is still insufficient evidence to determine the correct dosage for children. For adults, you can try it in tea, about 2-4 grams of soaked dried root or 1-2 teaspoons of whole or crushed berries soaked in about 2/3 cup of boiling water for 10-15 minutes three times a day. You can also take a tincture from 1/2 to 1 1/2 teaspoon three times a day or in the form of dry extracts about 250-500 milligrams three times a day.

Again, there are a few steps you need to consider. This drug has known problems when used with antibiotics, antihistamines, anticoagulants, blood pressure medications, diuretics, and diabetes medications, among others. Be sure to inform your doctor before trying any of the proposed doses.

The Hydra

Another Native American plant, the Canadian Hydra, was originally used for skin problems, digestive disorders, and irritated eyes. It has many medical uses today, including use as an antibiotic, immune booster, and treatment of upper respiratory tract problems (including sinuses).

Again, it is not recommended to use this herb for children. For adults, you can try capsules or tablets for 500-1000 mg up to three times a day, standardized extract in 30-120 mg, three times a day, or in the form of tincture (1:5): 2 - 3 mL, three times a day.

Do not take it if you are pregnant, breastfeeding, or have high blood pressure, liver, or heart problems without your doctor's consent. Interaction with anticoagulants is also known. Again, it is very important to inform your doctor if you plan to take this herb.

Eucalyptus

This native Australian and Tasmanian are widely used today as an alternative herb. It has antibacterial properties and acts as an expectorant that releases mucus into the body.

Again, be careful when using it with children. Children should never eat leaves or oil. Use only cough drops with eucalyptus in children older than six years.

For adults, you can try eucalyptus leaf as an infusion or tea about 1/4-1/2 teaspoon per cup of warm water, three times a day. Steep about 10-15 minutes and drink according to recommendations.

Consult your doctor before taking any of these medicines. All these tips can be found on the UMM site.

EVERYTHING YOU NEED TO KNOW ABOUT HERBS DETOXIFICATION

Herbal detoxification is known to cleanse the colon, skin, intestines, and other organs of the body. According to studies to be effective herbal antivirals, antiseptics, antibiotics, and antifungals to eliminate the harmful toxins in the body.

When your body is in full health, it can do its job correctly and effectively remove bad toxins. However, if the body is not well fed, and if you drink too much alcohol, no exercise, and various medications, your system may slow down and cause a blockage. You can use different types of herbs to detoxify your body to improve its metabolism and promote a healthy digestive system, with the aim to remove toxins and excess accumulated fluid from the body. However, before using any herbal preparations, it is necessary to consult a doctor.

Astragalus-this is one of the most common herbs that can be used alone or in combination with other herbs. It can help reduce the level of toxins in the liver, which will help improve mobility and increase blood flow. Astragalus is usually designed as a natural remedy for people with high blood pressure.

Aloe vera-This is an ancient medicinal herb that can help cleanse the large intestine. In order to get as much grass as possible, it is better to take it orally. It is known to be effective in the treatment of intestinal disorders and removes harmful toxins from the large intestine. Aloe vera contains anthranoids, which cleanses the intestines and promotes the healthy excretion of electrolytes and fluids in the intestines, causing a laxative effect for a period of about 9 hours. Because some of them may have undesirable side effects, such as heart arrhythmia, cramping, bone damage, and water retention, it is best to consult with your doctor before you start taking aloe vera.

Garlic is one of the most effective detoxifying herbs used for hundreds of years. Eating garlic, to a moderate degree, can help reduce cholesterol. It contains antifungal properties that can help cure yeast infections. However, it is important to note that consuming too much garlic can lead to possible adverse effects, such as fever, itching, runny nose, chills, sweating, and dizziness.

Cascara-this is a well-known bark laxative, which contains strong stimulants that can help with the evacuation of the intestine. It contains anthraquinones that can help promote colon contraction. However, there are possible side effects when used for a long time, such as the depletion of potassium and sodium, changing the color of the colon, abdominal cramps, hepatitis, and benign and cancerous growths. Pregnant women, nursing mothers, and people with gastrointestinal disorders, hemorrhoids, irritable bowel syndrome, and colitis should not take Cascara.

Dandelion leaves-helps to relieve the accumulation of fluid in tissues, stimulate excretion, and increase the amount of urine. This herb can be used in several ways; you can include them in your daily salad, steam the leaves, or use the dried leaves for tea. People taking pharmaceutical diuretics should consult their doctor before using the herb. Although no common side effects are expected, some people may develop a rash.

Detoxifying herbs are very effective, but due to the fact that herbs are powerful natural remedies, it should be used under the supervision of a physician.

Detoxification Herbal Formula

Most traditional detoxifying products contain herbs. The Detox Products that contain herbal extracts higher are able to restore health to an optimum level by increasing the efficiency of the removal of the organs in removing toxins, revitalizes your vigor, nourishes your body, strengthens the immune system, improves digestion, helps in weight loss and makes you look younger.

Below are the main types and functions of eight higher herbs that are able to help improve the effectiveness of the elimination organs in detoxification.

- Rhizoma Atractylodis Macrocephalae. (regulates bowel movement, spleen and improves vitality).

- Poria Cocos (removes toxins and improves skin condition)

- Radix cynanchum (removes toxins and reduces the number of fats)

- Radix Rubia Yunnanensis (improvement of blood circulation)

- Folium Nelumbo nucifera Gaertn (nourish the body)

- Radix Panax Quinguefolium (improve vitality)

- Gravel Root (helps to dissolve kidney stones and cleanse the kidneys)

- Folium Aloe Vera (an ingredient with a laxative effect, promotes better intestinal regulation, prevents constipation and destroys bacteria, viruses, yeasts and parasites in your system)

To facilitate swallowing, most of the herbal extracts in detoxification products are encapsulated and preferably taken with food for better digestion and absorption.

Detoxification is not for everyone. It is not recommended for patients with diabetes, liver problems, intestinal ulcer, cancer, and in patients treated with warfarin. People who are treated with any disease should consult their doctor before starting a special diet. Pregnant women, nursing mothers, and children should not follow a diet or a detoxification program. Do not immediately start a detoxification program if you suffer from fatigue, indigestion, cough, muscle aches, and poor sleep or other symptoms. Symptoms can be signs of a serious illness. It is important to consult your doctor for a thorough evaluation to make sure that these symptoms are not caused by a medical condition that requires immediate treatment.

It is necessary to remember that herbal dietary supplements are not the only effective means of detoxifying the body. You will also need exercise, rest, clean water, and a healthy diet. Remember that frequent detoxification improves your vitality, helps you feel better, and helps slow down the aging process.

HERBAL ANTIBIOTICS

Systemic Herbs

The following five herbs are very useful in the treatment of systemic infections, such as tuberculosis, malaria, MRSA, and Drug-Resistant Staphylococcus:

Cryptolepissanguinolenta

The root of the herb, Cryptolepis bloody, is used in traditional medicine in Africa to treat a number of diseases, such as jaundice, malaria, urinary tract infection, hepatitis, hypertension, stomach pain, and other inflammatory conditions. There is no evidence of toxicity, although the roots of this herb are consumed every day for years in the range. A number of interesting pharmacological properties are present in the raw extract and other components of the plant alkaloids. Dry extract of this herb is available in the form of teabags, which can be consumed every day. People in Ghana consumed it to avoid falciparum bacteria.

Acute AIDS

The leaves of acute aids are Oval, shredded, and cordate. On the fruit disc? The plant contains chlorides, alkaline sulfate, asparagines, ash, calcium carbonate, and magnesium phosphate. The roots of this plant are considered refreshing, fortifying, astringent, bitter, multiplying, antipyretic, and diuretic. It is often used to treat bacterial infections, fever, nervous system disorders, sciatica, facial paralysis, and promotes wound healing.

The preferred mode of consumption is a decoction; it is usually given to patients suffering from fever and occasional chills. Root juice is often used to accelerate the wound healing process. Powder of bark and root IU consumed by sugar and milk in the process of urination. Extremely useful oil is prepared with the addition of sesame oil and milk in the decoction of acute AIDS. This has a great impact on the treatment of disorders of the nervous system, sciatica, and facial paralysis. The leaves of the plant can be cooked and eaten to heal the bloody piles. A very important thing to understand here is the Ayurvedic concept of doshas. According to Ayurveda, there are three doshas: Vata, Pitta, and Kapha. The balance between the three doshas is necessary for optimal health. Acute AIDS is one of the few herbs that guarantee an optimal balance between three doshas.

Alchorneacordifolia

In the study of the leaves, stem, and bark of the roots of the plant alchorneacordifolia, it was found that the plants showed significant antimicrobial activity against Bacillus subtilis, Pseudomonas aeruginosa and Escherichia coli (or E. coli). It is an extremely effective herbal antibiotic that can provide the prevention and treatment of diseases.

"50% ethanol extract of alchorneacordifolia (Schum and Thonn) Muell. Argument. The Leaf was projected for activity against 74 microbial strains representing optional aerobic, and anaerobic bacteria and fungi. The panel of test strains included organisms from crop collections and clinical and environmental isolates. Concentration 5 mg / mL the extract inhibited 36.5% of isolates and 95.9% inhibited the concentration 20 mg / mL.only three strains, all filamentous fungi, were not sensitive to the 40 mg / mL extract, the highest Test concentration. The extract showed the best activity against gram-positive bacteria and yeast with inhibitory concentrations against these organisms at less than 5 mg/ml. The results show that the extract of A. cordifolia has a very wide spectrum of activity and suggests that it may be useful in the treatment of various microbial infections."

Hairy Bidens

Bidens pilosa, used as a medicinal plant in Africa, Asia, and tropical America. Leaves, roots, and seeds of narcotic, antibacterial, anti-inflammatory, antimalarial, antimicrobial, hepatoprotective, diuretic and hypotensive. Medically, the grass is used in five different ways:

- Sap from crushed leaves is used to accelerate the process of blood clotting in fresh wounds
- A decoction of leaves used to treat headaches
- The plant is used in the form of drops to treat ear infection
- Decoction with leaf powder is used to treat kidney problems
- And herbal tea made from the plant to eliminate bloating

Extracts from the plant, Bidens pilosa, have been used in South Africa to treat malaria. It is used in Zimbabwe to treat mouth and stomach ulcers, headaches, and diarrhea. The water that remained from the cooking of this herb is stored for this purpose. The suspension formed from the powder leaves is also used in an enema to treat abdominal discomfort. People in Congo use a mixture of the whole plant as a toxic antidote. They also use it to facilitate the birth process of a child and to greet the pain that comes out of the hernia. South Africans use decoctions of the plant to treat inflammatory conditions such as arthritis. The herb also finds use in the treatment of dysentery and jaundice. The plant can be used to treat burns. The powder obtained from seeds is used in the form of a local anesthetic for wounds and cuts. It is also used to treat spleen swelling in children. The plant, therefore, helps to fight bacteria, and is a powerful immune tonic, and is often used as an anti-inflammatory.

Annual Artemisia

It is a gently aromatic herb with small yellow buds and contains chemical artemisinin. Aerial parts of the plant are used in the production of antimalarial drugs. The plant is also called annual Wormwood. The herb has been used in traditional Chinese medicine to treat fever, jaundice, dizziness, headache, and nosebleeds. Chemical artemisinin is an extremely potent antimalarial drug. In fact, it can kill the deadliest parasite of malaria.

Non-Systemic Herbs

The next three herbs have a great effect on the treatment of urinary tract infections, gastrointestinal, and skin:

American Hydrastis

The root of the American Canadian hydrastis or Hydrastis Canadensis is appreciated as a stomach, tonic, and also used for use for sore eyes. It works very well in the case of general ulceration and has very vigorous measures against bacteria that cause food poisoning.G Salmonella and E. coli.

The mechanism of action is a laxative, tonic, and alterative. It is one of the best drugs for digestive disorders and shows them.

Special events on the mucous membrane. This makes it a valuable remedy for mucus. Herb has shown impressive results in the treatment of hemorrhoids and is used in chronic inflammation of the rectum and colon. It is administered in the form of injections to treat hemorrhoids with great success. Dried hydrastis nominal root powder used as a snuff for nasal mucus.

Grass is used for dyspepsia, loss of appetite, gastric mucus, and liver problems. It is an excellent gastric tonic for habitual constipation and an excellent remedy for vomiting and diseases.

It is used in tea as a decoction or infusion. It is also available in liquid form or in capsule form. Compresses are also used for local applications.

Juniper

Juniper grows in nature in parts of North America, Europe, and Asia. A short tree at medium height with the most popular variety is the Juniper communis. Juniper berries are used to make medicines. These include an extract of juniper berries and essential oil of the plant. Juniper has long been used for problems related to gastrointestinal tract like bloating, heartburn, stomach pain, bloating, loss of appetite, and intestinal worms. It is also used for Stones in the bladder and kidneys ATS

Good in urinary tract infections. It is hugely effective in the treatment of snake bites, cancer, and diabetes. Essential oil is often inhaled to treat bronchitis. Juniper not only reduces gases and inflammation but also fights with viruses and bacteria.

Usnea

Usnea is a variety of lichens that grow on trees. Although lichens resemble unique plants, they are an example of the symbiotic relationship between algae and fungi. They flourish in flat, colored spots. Usnea can be black, reddish, or whitish. The plant body of the herb is used for medicinal purposes.

Usnea is usually used generally to relieve pain, control weight, heal wounds, and control fever. It also helps to cure cough. It can be used on the skin of the mouth and throat in case of sore throat and ulcers in the mouth. The inflammation of the tonsils is extremely strong. The ingredients of the plant allow it to fight these bacteria and thereby fight infections.

Honey

Today, many people accept honey because of its anti-inflammatory and antibacterial properties. It is often considered one of the best complex drugs of nature by holistic professionals. Honey prevents the growth of pathogens such as salmonella and E.coli. It also fights against bacteria such as Pseudomonas aeruginosa and Staphylococcus aureus. You will notice that some types of honey are lighter, while some are darker. The one called the gift has better antioxidant and antibacterial abilities.

Synergistic Herbs

These herbs increase the activity of other herbs by increasing the number of antibacterial agents in the body, thereby improving the overall immune function.

Licorice

Licorice root with a long list of uses and makes it one of the most neglected herbal remedies. The main therapeutic compounds of the herb is called glycyrrhizin (and is at least fifty times sweeter than sugar), which is a valuable herb for treating a number of diseases. It is known that licorice increases the overall immune system in the body.

The listed benefits of grass include:

- Glycyrrhizic acid in licorice has great benefits in the treatment of anxiety, nervousness, and depression.
- Licorice root increases the flow of bile and eventually controls cholesterol levels by removing excess cholesterol from the body.
- Antiviral effect of the herb helps to treat herpes and shingles.
- Tablets and ointments based on grass are used to treat psoriasis, eczema, dry skin, and rashes.
- Calms the digestive system and helps with stomach problems.
- It is also used for weight reduction.
- Prevents gastrointestinal ulcers.
- Spasmodic, anti-inflammatory, and estrogenic effect and a great help for menstrual cramps, mood swings, bloating and nausea.
- It is useful in hormonal problems such as mood swings, exhaustion, and hot flashes.
- It is really useful in the treatment of polycystic ovarian disease.
- It is also an expectorant that takes place.

Instructions for use:

Licorice is best taken as a tea. To prepare this tea, the root of the grass is cut into thumbs and placed between layers of waxed paper. The pieces are then broken with sleds and powder prepared with a pestle and mortar. A teaspoon of this powder, and then put them in gauze and put in a bowl filled with boiling water. This can be soaked for about ten minutes and sweetened with honey.

Ginger

Pleasantly spicy, aromatic-ginger is often used as a special ingredient in Asian curries, fruit dishes, biscuits, and sweets. The ginger pulp can be white, yellow, or red depending on the variety used.

The listed benefits of grass include:

- Ginger contains zinc, magnesium, and chromium, which helps blood circulation and protection against fever, chills, and excessive sweating.
- It is an extremely powerful remedy for motion sickness.
- Improves the absorption of essential nutrients for the body.
- IME has a safe stroke treatment for flu and cold.
- Ginger also helps digestion.
- Reduces pain and inflammation.
- Helps fight respiratory problems such as cough and congestion.
- Protects against colorectal cancer.
- Ginger powder is known to trigger cell death in ovarian cancer cells.

- Strengthens immunity and fights morning sickness.

Instructions for use:

You can add two tablespoons of grated ginger to a cup of hot water to brew your healthy cup of tasty ginger tea. A teaspoon of honey not only softens tea but also helps to increase your immunity.

Freshly grated ginger can be combined with water, lemon juice, and brown sugar to prepare interesting and healthy lemonade

Just mix ginger, garlic, soy sauce, and olives for a healthy seasoning.

Your curry and sautéed can be seasoned with a teaspoon of grated ginger.

Pepper

Many people today consume black pepper. But they do not know that they subconsciously work to strengthen their immunity. Medicinal and consumed black pepper soothe stomach pain, cure bronchitis, and help in cancer. Antibacterial action makes it really useful to treat cholera and malaria. Anti-inflammatory action makes it a useful element in the treatment of scabies. It is used to relieve nerve pain.

Basil: Basil is often called the king of herbs due to the high presence of phytonutrients in the grass. In many countries around the world, it is also called "holy grass."

Basil

- Basil leaves have great benefits for Health Promotion and disease prevention.
- Polyphenolic flavonoids found in the herb provide incredible antioxidant benefits.
- The essential oils found in basil (e.g., eugenol, Linalool, terpineol, etc.) have excellent antibacterial and anti-inflammatory properties.
- Vitamin K in basil helps to strengthen bones.
- It is an excellent source of minerals such as copper, iron, magnesium, and manganese.
- Basil is a rich source of vitamin a, beta-carotene, lutein and cryptoxanthin, which is ideal for combating aging and maintaining good health

- Basil is also useful for arthritis and neuralgia.
- It can clean the sinuses and provide protection against colds and flu.

Instructions for use:

Basil oil can be used locally to help in cramps, rheumatism, and neuralgia.

A pinch of basil snuff is a great remedy for blocked breasts.

Do you suffer from blocked breasts and constipation? Don't worry! Just pour a little warm water on a teaspoon of basil powder and leave to infuse for ten minutes. Drink it while it's hot like herbal tea to feel immediate relief.

THE PRODUCTION OF MEDICINES

The preparation of medicines begins with the collection of plants, drying of the necessary parts, and subsequent storage for medical use. The first step in this process is to identify the plant you want to harvest. Then you should check the terrain around the area. In addition, you should not hear noise on a busy road, and you should not notice the fields of plants that are sprayed with pesticides.

The good harvest of plants ensures that they make fun of you in return! Now, if the plant is in good soil for harvesting, you can start the process of harvesting your plant.

Several methods are widespread for this purpose. Some people identify a large plant and call it a grandmother. They adore this grandmother and ask for permission to collect surrounding plants. In some cases, the process of collecting municipalities.

Always remember to collect with gratitude. That's because you force the plant to share its vitality with you, right? The best time to collect the aerial parts of the plant (including the leaf, stem, flower, and bark) and complete month. Similarly, those parts of the plant that are underground (necessarily the root) are best collected during the new moon.

The most favorable season for aerial harvesting parts is summer and spring, while the most favorable season for harvesting roots is late autumn or early spring.

The ideal time for harvesting would be in the early morning hours when the morning dew had already evaporated, and the sun was not strong enough to contain the plant. Always try to collect on a clear and sunny day.

You just need to collect the parts of the plant that you need. In the process, you want to choose only healthy portions. Therefore, you need to carefully choose healthy leaves and discard those contaminated with insects and moles. You can cut the entire stem or grow a new growth from above. This will also accelerate the growth of the plant. Do not forget to be extremely careful when harvesting roots, which leads to the death of the plant. Start by loosening the soil around the plant to extract the roots gently. The roots of the STEM can be a little heavy for harvesting and can also break during the process.

Always fill the soil with Earth once the roots are extracted.

The next logical step is to dry the plants, which will require special effort. Dry all aerial parts of the plant in bundles small enough to allow optimal air circulation. You can hang plants on the ropes; they must be suspended in a place where they receive optimal air circulation and are not exposed to direct sunlight. Leaves, stems, bark, and flowers can be dried in nylon baskets. Metal baskets are strict, "no."

The roots of the plant should be thoroughly washed before trying to dry them. Now you can cut them into small pieces, wash them, and then dry them, put them in baskets. It is necessary to store all dried herbs in airtight containers (preferably glass).You can carefully mark the jars and store them in a cool, dry place away from direct sunlight.

Now that you understand the process of harvesting, drying, and storing your plants, let's look at the process of creating the drug.

Preparation of Herbal Teas

You can prepare your herbal tea in the process of decoction or infusion. Decoctions can extract the healing properties of bark, roots, fungi, and other hard surfaces. To get the perfect broth, you need to grind or grate part of the plant. However, this process may require a little extra effort. You need to break the large pieces of the plant into small pieces, and then grate them into pieces in a stainless steel or glass pan. It should be covered with cold water and then brought to a boil. Boil by putting on the stove. The flame should be reduced when the water begins to boil, and the solution should be cooked on low heat for about forty minutes. The solution should be kept overnight in a warm state.

Infusions can extract the healing properties of the stem, leaves, bark, flowers, and even some roots. Dry plants rub in your hands, and fresh; you can simply tear or chop. This process begins the release of essential oils from plants, destroying the cell walls of the plant. Herbs should be placed in a stainless steel or glass container and poured with boiling water. The container should be covered only that the medicinal substances of this tea do not fall off with the steam.

Solar infusion extracts the healing properties of the grass with the help of the sun. You can keep the grated grass covered, pour water into a glass jar, and put it in the sun. Lunar infusion, aimed at extracting the healing properties of the grass from it by taking the help of the Moon. Herbs should be poured with water and kept in the moonlight. The choice of the container is extremely important. Always choose stainless steel, glass, or enamel containers during the process of creating decoctions and infusions. Plastic and aluminum containers can react with plants and therefore cause more harm than benefit.

You can rotate them as much as you want (depending on the power you want). However, some plants, such as chamomile, can become bitter if left for a long time. On the other hand, there are plants such as Nettles that can be infused overnight. It also makes them richer in minerals!

The most important thing to remember in the process of preparing such teas is your intention and the power of positive statements. You just have to think about all the positive changes you want to welcome into your life and release energy from your water-filled plant to fill you with energy, vitality, and good health. It should also be remembered that vegetable water evaporates during drying. Therefore, dried plants are more concentrated than fresh ones. Here is a basic dosage guide for use in medical teas:

Dry herbs: infusions and decoctions can be prepared with a tablespoon of dry herbs on a glass of water.

Fresh herbs: the dosage for the use of fresh herbs will be twice as high as for dry ones. Therefore, a glass of water will need two tablespoons.

Preparation of Tincture

Tinctures are concentrated liquid extracts based on medicinal herbs. Liquid, which is used to obtain the healing properties of herbs, is called menstruation. Examples of menstruation are alcohol, glycerin, and vinegar.

Tinctures can be consumed with water or diluted in water, tea, or juice. Adding the tincture to a glass of extremely hot water ensures that the alcohol from the tincture evaporates before use.

To prepare tinctures, you can use a number of methods. I usually prepare my own dried herbal tinctures and let them absorb in the menstruation of at least one full moon. To prepare tinctures, the plants are ground and poured into a clean jar, leaving little room for menstruation. Add a little water before adding the last menstrual cycle. Mix everything together. Now, pour menstruation and tightly close the lid. Keep this for two weeks. Shake the mixture every day, and once you are sure of the desired strength (about two weeks later),strain the mixture, compressing each piece of medicinal plant. Pour it into amber bottles and store it in a cool, dry place.

Ointment Preparation

The mixture of herbs, oils, and wax applied to the skin from the outside is called ointment. Ointments protect the skin and are often used with extreme dryness, bites, rashes, rashes, burns, fungi, etc. However, the most popular method of cooking includes a warming cup of vegetable oil in a frying pan. Add about five tablespoons of chopped beeswax, let the oil warm-up. Continue to stir constantly. The mixture should be placed in containers and stored in the freezer when it hardens. You can also pour additional ingredients, such as essential oils or vitamin E, before wrapping the fat in containers. The shelf life of fat is usually years. They last longer if they are put in a cool, dark place.

Here are some possible fats and balms:

- Mint chocolate lip balm can be made using peppermint oil and peppermint essential oil.
- Anti-fat can be prepared using herbs such as eucalyptus, rosemary, thyme, or mint.
- Antifungal ointment is prepared from herbs, such as essential oils of the tea tree and calendula flowers.
- Therapeutic ointment is used from plants such as St. John's wort and flowers.

Floor Preparation and Low-Temperature Brazing, High-Temperature Brazing

So, it's very simple. To prepare a compress, you simply need to moisten a clean cloth in a herbal decoction, infusion, or tincture. And pots can be made from a paste of dried plants and mixed with water. It is then heated to a temperature that the skin can withstand. I hope you enjoyed reading this book and make sure you live a wonderful life without the use of pharmaceutical antibiotics and antiviral drugs. It will not only help you get rid of the antibiotic resistance to which your body is accustomed but will also bring you to a healthier and happier state!

Manufactured by Amazon.ca
Bolton, ON